THE HOME
HERBAL DOCTOR

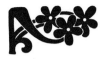
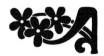

THE HOME
HERBAL DOCTOR

HOWARD H. HIRSCHHORN

Parker Publishing Company, Inc.
West Nyack, New York

Fourth Printing . . . . . September 1987

Library of Congress Cataloging in Publication Data

Hirschhorn, Howard H.
  The home herbal doctor.

  Includes index.
    1. Herbs—Therapeutic use.   2. Medicine—
Formulae, receipts, prescriptions.   3. Therapeutics
—Popular works.   I. Title.
  RM666.H33H57   615'.321   82-6490

ISBN 0-13-392837-3
ISBN 0-13-392829-2 {PBK}   AACR2

Printed in the United States of America

Foreword

Today's market offers a plethora of books on "nature's medicines"—some reliable and based on sound research, many of dubious trustworthiness and questionable basis. Howard H. Hirschhorn's contribution is not just another book on plant medicines: it is conceived and written from a novel point of view.

Medicinal plants usually owe their biodynamic activity to their chemical content. Consequently, an understanding of the active principles of the medicine should take high priority in any consideration of therapeutically used members of the Plant Kingdom. Hirschhorn's emphasis is on the chemical makeup of the plants which he takes up in 12 sections.

As the author brings out in several places, the activity of some of the plants which experience has proven to be biodynamic—alleviating or relieving unpleasant symptoms—cannot always be attributed to the known chemical constitution. But in these few cases, he intimates that more research might be warranted. While written in a popular style, this book brings together a wealth of information, much of it thought-provoking for investigators interested in further research.

The appeal to a wide audience of Hirschhorn's novel method of approach will assure this volume an interested and broad market and should be welcomed as a significant contribution to ethnopharmacology.

Richard Evans Schultes, Ph. D.
Professor of Biology and
Director, Botanical Museum
of Harvard University,
Cambridge, Massachusetts

How Practical Experience plus Scientific Probing Reveal the Health Powers of Plants

Explorers and other travelers once reported that Andean Indians sprinkled powdered plantain or ribgrass leaf on poorly healing sores to speed up healing, just as European farmers and U.S. settlers did. The Andean Indians and some European farmers still do it today. And today, lavender flowers relieve headaches and sleeplessness in the Andes, just as they do in many other places in the world; lavender was most likely relieving those headaches in South America long before Europeans ever heard of the Americas. These and many more apparent coincidences in the use of the same plants for the same ailments in different parts of the world can be amazing proof of the properties of those plants ... even before modern science gets around to verify them. In quite a few cases, scientific research does verify that a plant has a certain effect, but cannot always give a reason for *why* or *how* that effect takes place ... and takes place it surely does, to our good fortune. To deny that is almost like refusing to let anyone have a baby until scientists can prove exactly what makes a baby by making one in a test tube first!

On the other hand, scientists have been able to find new uses for old plants once the ingredients—the natural chemicals—of the plant were identified. Those ingredients can often be extracted and concentrated for use as a safe, effective and economical medicine. In other cases, however, the plant's natural ingredients can unfold and develop their effects only as part of the whole plant ... in the natural company of other ingredients in the plant where all these chemical ingredients were formed all together by the miraculous natural chemistry of the tiniest of factories—a plant that lives on earth, sun and water.

This book tells about many curative plants whose benefits to health have already been proven by centuries, in many cases, of successful use. And this use was not only by practical-minded rural folk who "know well what they know," but also by highly trained and experienced physicians and pharmacists. Almost every plant and/or remedy in this book, in fact, has been approved for public use and sale by health and medical authorities in various countries whose scientific and medical traditions are, without doubt, world renowned. In short, botanical or herbal medicine is definitely one of our essential, natural weapons against ill health; some plant substances, as remedies, alleviate and even cure disease; other plant substances, as part of a good diet, actually prevent disease and maintain good health. (You can easily prove this by not taking enough of it, then seeing what happens to you!). This book reports how such plant remedies have been used and still are being used in the service of good health.

Howard H. Hirschhorn

Contents

Section 1

The Natural Chemicals in Plants and Their Startling Effects on Your Health

Many of the plants from which we can prepare comforting and even healing teas, baths, dressings, wines and other remedies for alleviating our ills are no strangers to the average kitchen. Sage, cinnamon, laurel or bay, caraway, anise, cardamon, thyme, onions, limes and lemons are only a very few of them.

Fine chefs who call onion an indispensable perfume would be happy to know that onion can dissolve away dangerous blood clots in the bood vessels of people who eat it regularly. Limes, of course, once saved Britania's Royal Navy from scurvy when her vitamin C-starved sailors were dropping out on long voyages. Ask any British sailor today, and he'll tell you it's true, for that's how he got the nickname *limey*.

Other plants, though not eaten regularly as food, can be taken regularly as tonics or protectors against disease and poor body function that can lead eventually to disease. Still other plants can be called upon occasionally when needed to alleviate pain and illness. Despite the flood of synthetic drugs, many properly extracted and combined plant substances are still among the best sources of safe, natural, effective and economical medicines.

15 natural plant chemicals that cure, protect and alleviate

Science attempts to pin down each effect of a plant by proving the existence of a specific active ingredient that is clearly responsible for the effect. This is often possible, but not always. Scientists cannot yet associate some effects with any particular active ingredient in some plants. But that lack of a scientific reason doesn't stop the effect from happening and being definitely verified by even the most sceptical scientists and physicians, who are, however, at a loss to explain *why* and *how*. It's believed that the *whole* plant with *all* of its ingredients is responsible for some effects. One inactive and apparently "useless" ingredient may temper another, overly active ingredient so as to let the remedy develop its best curative or protective powers, but not its strongest effects. Raspberries are an example of how ingredients affect one another. Raspberries contain more fruit acids than currants contain, but don't taste as sour as currants. That's because the mucilage in raspberries takes the edge off the acidity.

Parts or extracts of several plants can be combined to develop the greatest safe curative power possible from them. An ingredient of one plant may release the active ingredient of another plant, or even reinforce its effect.

One convenient way to classify the active ingredients of medicinal plants is chemically—the plants in each natural chemical group showing similar and predictable effects on us. *Important note: a plant can belong to more than one group.* Mullein, for example, is both a saponin-containing expectorant (which gets phlegm up) and a polysaccharide-containing demulcent (that is, its mucilage soothes issues); both properties are good for respiratory conditions.

On the other hand, different parts of the same plant can have different effects: tannin-containing dried blueberries stop diarrhea, and arbutin-containing blueberry leaves disinfect urinary passages.

Even the same part of a plant can have different effects: *fresh* blueberries are laxative, but *dried* blueberries stop diarrhea.

Group 1—phlegm-loosening saponins

Saponins get their name from the Latin word for *soap* because they foam if you shake them in water. "Soap plants" have been, and still are, used by native peoples in various parts of the world.

Saponins speed up the passage of other substances through the walls of the gastrointestinal tract and stimulate secretion from the mammary glands and from some of the glands along the respiratory tract.

Examples of saponin-containing plants that act as expectorants, that is, help get phlegm up and out, are primrose or cowslip roots, lungwort leaves, and mullein flowers and leaves.

Examples of saponin-containing plants that act as diuretics, that is, increase the flow of urine, are Java tea leaves and goldenrod foliage.

Examples of saponin-containing plants that help re-establish the smooth functioning of body fluids and forces are pansy foliage and horsetail foliage.

Saponin-containing goat's rue or galega stimulates lactation in nursing mothers.

Group 2—disinfectant and pain-relieving phenolglycosides

Arbutin, one of the phenolglycosides, has a disinfecting action on the urinary tract when the urine is alkaline. Bearberry leaves and blueberry leaves are examples of arbutin-containing plants.

Salicin, another phenolglycoside, reduces fever and relieves articular rheumatism. Salicin is related chemically to the salicylic acid in aspirin, and thus provides some of the pain-relieving and fever-reducing properties of aspirin. Meadowsweet foliage, pansy foliage, willow bark, and poplar leaves and bark are examples of plants that contain salicin.

Group 3—bowel-moving anthraglycosides

Anthraquinone, also called emodin, is one of the anthraglycosides that relieves constipation. Senna leaves, aloes, buckthorn bark, and rhubarb are examples of plants that contain anthraquinone or emodin.

Group 4—cardiovascular-active flavonoids

Flavonoids get their name from the Latin *flavus* for yellow because flavonoid derivatives are yellow, at least in the chemist's test tube if not in the plant. Some flavonoids exert favorable effects on the heart; others affect the kidneys so as to promote the flow of urine; still others can inhibit infections. Rutin, one of the flavonoids, has an anti-hemorrhagic effect which keeps blood from leaking out of the circulatory system's smallest blood vessels, the capillaries. Rutin also helps blood vessels to expand, leading to lower blood pressure. Examples of flavonoid-containing plants are hawthorn flowers, broom foliage, birch leaves, linden blossoms, juniper berries, and camomile flowers.

Group 5—antibiotic and circulation-improving mustard oils

Plants that contain mustard oil glycosides may be used as rubifacients, that is, they redden the skin, improving circulation of the blood near the surface. Mustard seed is familiar to all who have ever used a mustard plaster to chase bronchitic distress and colds, or who have ever heard their grandmothers talk about it. Mustard oil glycosides also act antibiotically, such as those in watercress.

Group 6—soothing anti-irritants and starches diabetics can eat

The polysaccharides include mucilage, pectin, starch, gums, and inulin. Mucilage soothes inflamed mucous membranes by reducing irritation and irritability of nerve endings, and by taking up harmful substances that would otherwise penetrate the tissues and harm them. Pectin, such as in apples, controls diarrhea and bleeding. Inulin, such as from elecampane roots, has been baked into bread for diabetics, who have little to fear from the fructose which results from the digestion of inulin. Fructose is readily metabolized in the body and is converted into glycogen ("animal starch") even when insulin is lacking. Examples of plants that contain mucilage are linseed or flaxseed, marshmallow root, coltsfoot leaves, Iceland moss, lance-leaf plantain, and all parts of mullein.

Group 7—anesthetic prussic acid

Prussic acid's local anesthetic effect and mucilage's soothing, protective effect are combined when a poultice of crushed linseed is applied to the skin, say on an ulcer. Almonds, too, contain prussic acid, which may be one of the reasons for the relief afforded when almond "milk" (almond oil shaken up with water) or almond oil is rubbed into chapped, cracked skin; the oil's soothing action, of course, also contributes.

Group 8—lifesaving heart glycosides

Leaves of the purplish-flowered foxglove contain digitalis glycoside, lily of the valley contains convallatoxin glycoside, pheasant's eye contains adonitoxin glycoside, and oleander contains oleandrin. These natural chemical compounds seem to have a particular affinity for exhausted heart muscle. Note the *toxic* part of some of the names, revealing that these powerful and lifesaving substances are only for experienced and cautious use, including the plants without the specific reference to *toxin* in their scientific names.

Group 9—antithrombotic coumarin

Perhaps the best known effect of coumarin is the sweet clover disease of cattle. In this disease, a coumarin derivate in the hay fodder can cause excessive bleeding in cattle if, for one reason or another, they have to be operated on. This effect, however, has been used medically to prevent or dissolve blood clots or thrombotic plugs in people. Woodruff and the toothpick or ammi plant are two other examples of coumarin-containing plants.

Group 10—astringent and antimicrobial tannins

You *tan* animal skins into leather with *tannis*, which also exert a very mild, medically useful version of tanning on our mucous membranes and skin ... where we think of it not as tanning, but as an astringent and tightening effect. Tannins also disinfect by destroying harmful microorganisms and by inhibiting decomposition. In addition, tannins combat diarrhea. Examples of plants that contain tannins are walnut leaves, tormentil rhizome, sage leaves, blueberries, and oak bark.

Group 11—digestion-promoting bitters

Bitters promote bile secretion and/or flow, improve the uptake of nutrients from the gastrointestinal tract, and stimulate digestive juices for improved digestion and better appetite (but not in people with normal appetites, so don't be afraid of eating yourself overweight). Bitters also combat gastrointestinal fermentation. Examples of plants that contain bitters are gentian root, angelica root, milfoil foliage, and wormwood foliage. These four plants are called *aromatic* bitters because they also contain ethereal (*or* aromatic *or* essential *or* volatile) oils, which are discussed next.

Group 12—ethereal oils that reduce inflammation, relieve cramping, promote milk flow, aid digestion, expel gas, disinfect, bring up phlegm, and calm the nerves

These plants give off their ethereal (also called aromatic, essential or volatile) oils when heated. Often, however, their characteristic odor is noticeable even without heating. Anise and other kitchen spices are examples. The properties of ethereal oils include the relief of gas and cramping, antiseptic and anti-inflammatory effects, promotion of the secretion and/or flow of body fluids (urine, bile, milk), improvement of digestion, getting phlegm up and out, and soothing the nerves. At least eight different effects, for example, are due to the ethereal oils in the four plants on the chart on p. 17.

Group 13—alkaloids with many beneficial characteristics

Alkaloids are nitrogen-containing compounds with certain chemical characteristics, such as reacting chemically like alkaline substances, and that's why they're called *alka*-oids (*oids* means *like*). Nicotine in tobacco is an alkaloid. Morphine and codeine in opium are well known pain-relieving alkaloids. Boldo leaves and Scotch broom contain spartein, an alkaloid that counters the effect of snake venom. The study of plant alkaloids is quite extensive, and it's very hard, if not impossible, to pin down a characteristic that fits all of them.

	Reduce inflammation	Relieve cramping	Promote milk flow	Expel gas	Disinfect	Bring up phlegm	Promote digestion	Calm nerves
Camomile flowers	YES	YES		YES	YES			YES
Melissa leaves		YES	YES	YES	YES			YES
Anise fruit ("seeds")		YES	YES	YES	YES	YES	YES	
Peppermint leaves	YES	YES		YES	YES	YES	YES	

Group 14—stimulating and heart-protecting purines

Caffeine—an example of a purine in coffee, maté tea, Chinese tea, and certain other teas—increases the flow of urine and supports healthy heart function ... even though too much of some of them may overstimulate and excite you so much that you feel as if your heart's running away with you.

Group 15—essential minerals

Plants, of course, contain minerals in addition to any of the other substances mentioned in the above sections. That's why we tell the kids to "eat all your vegetables ... they'll make you strong ... make you grow ... give you rosy cheeks ..." And it's true, for many plants contain very large amounts of one or several minerals, depending upon the soil and growing conditions. Spinach, for example, contains a large amount of iron as well as vitamin A and other valuable, even vital, substances. Popeye was nobody's dummy—he knew how to turn into a man of iron by eating spinach! Horsetail is rich in silicon, a mineral shown to clear up the symptoms of arteriosclerosis in rats. Fucus or bladder wrack seaweed, rich in iodine, has been used to treat people who suffered from certain forms of goiter and has also been eaten by obese people (as long as they didn't also suffer from a hyperthyroid condition) to increase their activity so they could reduce·

Preparation of teas, rinses, and baths

The simplest *general* rule for making teas (also called *infusions* if brewed or steeped, and *decoctions*, if hard parts are boiled), rinses, and baths are:

1. For soft parts such as flowers and leaves, pour 1 cupful of boiling water over 1 teaspoonful of the crushed dried plant material and steep 5 minutes in a covered cup before straining. Drink warm·

2. For hard parts such as roots, bark, seeds and seed-like fruit (like anise "seeds"), boil 1 teaspoonful of the crushed or powdered dry plant material in 1 cupful of water for 3 to 5 minutes. Strain. Drink warm·

3. Use porcelain (fireproof) glass or other non-reactive containers such as coated or stainless-steel ones if porcelain and glass are unavailable.

4. Don't overheat plant parts from which you want ethereal oils, for too much heat drives them off (that's why they're called *volatile* oils ... they escape into the air). Some teas or infusions are made without any heat at all, such as marshmallow root, which is soaked about 6 hours to extract the mucilage. Some plant ingredients are not easily soluble in water, and are extracted with other solvents such as medical-grade drinking alcohol (ethyl alcohol), brandy, or wine. Most of the remedies described in this book can be brewed as teas or baths ... but they can also be obtained in professionally prepared tonics and tinctures (some of which I've enjoyed as health-promoting holiday spirits!) as well as in genuine alcoholic beverages not usually consumed primarily for their herbal content, such as angelica-containing *Chartreuse*, artichoke (cynarin)-containing

Cynara, and gentian-containing *Enzian*—gentian schnaps. But that shouldn't surprise us, for alcohol did begin as a medicine, not as a beverage.

Below is a table of guidelines just a bit more detailed than the above very general rules:

Condition of plant parts	Fresh or dried. Some plant parts are best if fresh (such as some vitamin-C-rich fruits). Some parts must be dried (such as buckthorn bark, which is stored 1 to 2 years to allow chemical changes to occur).
Soft and/or light parts (flowers, foliage or whole herb, flowering tops, stems, leaves, soft fruit, sap)	To brew a tea or infusion for drinking, wet compresses, or addition to baths, pour 1 *cupful* boiling water (some people use the official 8-ounce cooking measure, and some use various sizes of tea or coffee cup or mug), over *1 teaspoonful* (from 2 to 4 grams) of the crumbled, crushed, grated or powdered dry plant part in a non-metallic (or non-reactive metal) container. *Steep 5 minutes* (some steep as few as 2 or 3, and others as much as 10 or 15 minutes). Drink hot (if you're sweating out colds with, say, elder or linden tea), lukewarm (most people drink most teas like this), or cool (some people find coolness more soothing in certain conditions. Certain plants taste better cold, such as senna).
Hard and/or dense parts (roots, rhizomes, inner bark, root bark, vines, nuts, seeds, seed-like fruits)	Use the same quantities as for the soft parts given above. Put the plant material in the water and bring it to a boil, then remove the whole pot from the heat and let it steep about 5 minutes (some do it 3 minutes and some as long as 30 minutes) before straining out and discarding the plant parts. Or, bring to boil and keep boiling until about 1/3 of the water has evaporated, then steep a few minutes before straining.

If the amount of heat described in the table above is still too much for a particular plant from which you want to brew a tea, then you can soak the parts in cold water. Marshmallow root, for example, may be soaked in cold water overnight to extract the mucilage ... strands of which you can see dangling from the floating chips of marshmallow root even after 30 to 45 minutes of soaking time.

Appropriate details for brewing teas and preparing rinses, douches, wet dressings, and baths are given throughout the book.

About medications in general

As a general rule, be wary of all unknown or unaccustomed medicines and remedies, especially excessive amounts of them, whether from your doctor's office, the corner drugstore, or from your own garden. If you are already on prescription or other medication, check with your physician before you take different medicines together. Physicians with herbal knowledge and experience usually advise their patients that teas, etc., work best when all other drugs (including coffee, for example) have cleared out of your body before you start to take herbal remedies.

Section 2

Over 100 Often-Used Plants, Many with Surprising Healing Properties Verified by Modern Science

These one hundred some plants are only a small part of the whole armory of weapons we have accumulated over the centuries in our battle against disease and ill health. *Battle*, however, is not always the best word for really effective and safe plant remedies that work *with* our physiology, not against it, in strengthening our resistance as well as actually alleviating disease and freeing us from unnecessary distress and pain. In quite a few cases, herbal remedies, as well as other of the natural methods of healing at our disposal, *orchestrate* our forces and physical resources into a well-coordinated functional whole which has the best possible opportunity of benefiting fully from our own individual health potential. All of these plants have helped someone before. Not all of the people all of the time, but many people many times.

**How a pharmacist grows a tropical
remedy during the winter at home for
relieving burns and constipation**

An Indian pharmacist from the island of Goa continued to grow his favorite remedy plant, aloe (*Aloe vera* and other species), even when he moved to Germany. Because of the radical change in climate, however, he grew his aloe indoors in Germany, instead of outside in the garden, as he did in his tropical homeland.

21

He cut open a fresh succulent leaf and used the jelly-like sap directly on insect stings and bites, burns (including sunburn) and other skin wounds and infections, just like Alexander the Great of Macedonia did (after he followed the advice of Aristotle to conquer the island of Socotra so as to have a steady supply of aloe) for treating his wounded soldiers. Also, the pharmacist brewed tea from the dried sap and used it to rinse out wounds.

For constipation, he stirred two ounces of aloe leaf pulp or jelly-like sap (fresh or in dried chunks) into twenty ounces of boiling water. Then he let the solution stand quietly for twenty-four hours, after which he poured off (and saved) the liquid, leaving the sediment and undissolved material behind, and then strained out the remaining debris floating in the liquid. The final step was to evaporate the liquid either in the sun or an oven, but not any hotter than 140°F. He used one to four grains (or about sixty to 250 milligrams) of the dried residue left behind after evaporation, but always took it with anti-gas and anti-cramping plants to counteract the griping and colic that sometimes accompanies aloe's laxative effect. (The Karanga of Africa drink aloe leaf juice in water to alleviate constipation *and* colic.) The physician for whom the Indian pharmacist made the aloe remedy didn't give it to any patients suffering from gastrointestinal irritation, or to pregnant or nursing mothers.

Although some people find that aloe tastes somewhat nauseating, it's not as bad as you'd be led to believe by the report made by South African farmers that a teaspoonful of concentrated aloe leaf juice given by mouth to a horse temporarily makes the animal's blood so bitter that any ticks on it drop off. But the taste is obviously distinctive, judging from the practice of Zulu and Chagga mothers in Africa of rubbing the leaf pulp over their breasts and nipples to speed up weaning their infants, who apparently don't like the taste.

The Zulu, Xhosa, Sotho and other African peoples use aloe leaf juice to relieve eye infections and inflammations. A Cuban nursery-man I met in Miami swallowed a pinch of dried aloe pulp to loosen up his occasional constipation. A Key Largo yachtswoman picked up a hot-handle griddle from her boat's galley, and felt it sizzle into her flesh. She dropped the griddle and reached for a fresh aloe leaf, holding the gelatinous pulp on her burned hand for 30 minutes, during which time her pain subsided. No blisters formed nor did any scars remain from that griddle burn.

I asked a Key West (Florida) aloe laboratory about the best way of growing aloe indoors in the U.S., and they recommended the following:

1. Aloe (*Aloe vera*) loves humidity but hates wet roots. Prolonged exposure to water-soaked soil rots the roots and kills the plant.

2. Aloe likes a loose, alkaline, well-drained soil. A light fertilizer every six months encourages growth.

3. Aloe, a tropical plant, can take hard sun but prefers some shade. Browning generally indicates too little water under heavy sun. Wilting generally means too much water.

4. The larger the pot the larger the plant. The root system grows horizontally a few inches below the surface of the soil, and needs spreading room to develop fully.

5. Small shoots develop from the "running root." When these young speckled shoots are about six inches high, they can be potted to begin a new plant. This repotting also helps the "mother" plant to develop more fully.

6. Be careful to remove only outer leaves of the aloe so as to avoid destroying its central growth core.

7. Under field conditions, aloe leaves can be harvested in three to five years.

8. In summary: water lightly, drain well, fertilize occasionally, and if all else fails, speak to it!

The aloe species in this section are not the same as the flowering or spiked aloe, which is really an agave (*Agave americana*).

How a farmer's wife flavors a cake with a plant that aids digestion, sleep, and nerves

Angelica or holy ghost plant (*Angelica archangelica*) may get its name from the beautiful and coquettish daughter, Angelica, of an ancient king of Cathay. The second part of angelica's scientific name, *archangelica* may refer to its superbly angelic properties, long recognized by the good monks of Chartreuse, who employed it to make their famous liqueurs. On the other hand, however, *archangelica* could also refer to the Russian port of Archangelsk, from where the plant has often been exported to the rest of the world. Scholars can't seem to agree on such things, but the theories do tell us some things about the plant's use and history, or at least that it was around while the history was being made. That's part of why I've mentioned the origin of plant names in this book. Another reason is that a plant's name may also describe the plant.

As a tea, angelica's ethereal oils, bitters, tannins, coumarin derivates, and other ingredients in its leaves and roots all contribute to preventing or overcoming gastritis, colic and cramping, gas, heartburn or indigestion, poor appetite, and nervous insomnia. Angelica also helps loosen mucoid secretions and encourages urinary flow. It may, however, also increase the amount of sugar in the blood of some people.

A central European farmer rubbed angelica liniment into his skin to allay the aches of rheumatism, gout, and neuralgia, and his wife sugared the leaf stalks of angelica for decorating her cakes, thus helping her family's digestion at the same time they were enjoying her cake.

The ethereal oil vapors that emanate from a small pillowcase stuffed with angelica foliage, and perhaps a few other aromatic plants, can calm the nerves and help a nervous insomniac fall asleep.

A spice that alleviated a
shipper's asthma and gas

In 1305 Edward I of England helped pay for repairs on London Bridge by including anise (*Pimpinella anisum*) among the items for which toll was to be exacted. So, like many useful plants, anise has been around awhile. The tranquilizing power of anise has long been utilized by European pigeon fanciers, who rub it on the walls of their pigeon lofts to accustom new birds to the strange surroundings; the aromatic odor of anise soon quietens the restless pigeons. Anise soothes cramping; it helps relieve stomach cramps and alleviate asthma, which owes part of its unpleasantness to cramping or tightening of the bronchial tubes. The ethereal oils in anise act favorably on the mucous membranes, especially of the digestive and respiratory systems, where the oils stimulate the ciliated cells to sweep better with their whip-like hairs so as to rid the respiratory passages of irritants. Anise's oils raise total metabolism, increase lagging secretions such as milk in nursing mothers, and enhance sexual prowess.

Star or Chinese anise (*Illicium verum* from China, other parts of Asia, and Jamaica) is also a source of anise oil. Japanese or bastard star anise (*Illicium anisatum* or *Illicium religiosum*), however, contains a toxic substance, and is not used in herbal remedies.

To alleviate or forestall his asthmatic attacks, the director of a London ship chandlery drank a cup or so of warm anise tea made by boiling crushed aniseed 10 minutes in 1 pint of water. The tea, when drunk just before he felt the attack coming on, reduced the severity of the impending attack. After mild attacks started, asthmatic discomfort usually abated after 1 to 2 cups of tea. He was so pleased with the additional benefits of his anise tea—its anti-gas and digestion-promoting effects—which he noticed whenever he drank the anise tea for his asthma, that he mixed up the following anise cordial for his dinner guests: he added 30 grams of crushed aniseed (the "seed" is the fruit of anise, but it's often called *aniseed*) plus 30 grams of crushed fennel "seed" (which is the seed-like fruit of fennel) plus 1 teaspoonful of malt sugar plus some lemon peel to 1 quart of good brandy.

In the Arab world, the fumes from a handful of aniseed thrown into a wood fire have been inhaled to alleviate dizziness and headaches. A North African merchant eased his "hiccoughing indigestion" by drinking a tea brewed from anise, lemon balm (melissa) leaves, and peppermint leaves. Also, this same merchant said he sparked up his sex life by eating a confection made from anise, stinging nettle seeds (*Urtica pilulifera*), cloves, and fennel.

How a pharmacist soothed bruises and sprains with a cardiovascular-active yellow flower

Arnica, mountain tobacco or wolf's bane (*Arnica montana*), may be named after the Greek word *arnakis* (sheep's or lamb's skin), referring to the woolly leaves and stems of the plant. Or the name may come from the Greek word *ptarmika* for *sneezeweed* because arnica can make you sneeze. On closed wounds and hemorrhoids, arnica reduces inflammation, acts antiseptically, relieves pain, helps clear up bleeding under bruised skin, and fosters healing.

Because arnica widens blood vessels, relieves cramping and generally stimulates circulation, it has been useful (but only under medical supervision) in alleviating or preventing angina pectoris, coronary sclerosis, coronary insufficiency, high blood pressure, asthma, and inflammed veins. Arnica may not be a cure-all, but it is definitely a "cure-a-lot." *As a home remedy, however, arnica should only be used externally*, such as in wet compresses or as a tincture to be daubed on closed wounds and bruises.

If your particular wound doesn't tolerate arnica, however, marigold tea as wet compresses or made into a tincture may be a better choice of a remedy.

A pharmacist from a town near Salzburg, Austria, made arnica tincture by collecting the flowers with or without foliage, cleaning them by picking out any soil particles, rinsing them off under cool, running water, and putting them in a clear glass bottle filled with ethyl alcohol (or a good brandy will do just fine, too). Then he left the filled bottle exposed to the warmth of the sun for ten days. Finally, the pharmacist strained out the plant parts and used the tincture on sprains, bruises, swellings, and areas affected by rheumatism. For use on minor cuts and scrapes he first diluted the arnica tincture by mixing 3 tablespoonsful of it with 1 quart of boiled water, then daubed that on the wounds.

Because of arnica's "cure-a-lot" reputation in the Alpine region where I recently spent the better part of a year on a research trip, I've compared two equally reputable arnica tinctures made by two different laboratories located right in that geographical area. (Both of them, by the way, are within a stone's throw from officially authorized medical spas where mineral springs and earths, herbals, and other natural healing methods are in everyday use to alleviate health problems.*)

---

*Many of these methods are described in *Miracle Health Secrets from the Old Country* Parker Publishing Company.

	Laboratory A (Dr. Otto Greither)	Laboratory B (Josef Mack)
Content	Every 10 grams of alcohol (a medical quality alcohol) contains 1.667 grams of arnica flowers	1 part arnica flowers to 3 parts ethyl alcohol (a medical quality alcohol)
Used for	Bruises, sprains, bleeding under the skin, abrasions, minor cuts. Irritated vocal cords and/or laryngitis.	Sprains and strains, bruises, bleeding under the skin, swellings, rheumatic distress, inflammed nerves (neuritis), inflammed tendons (tendonitis) arthritis, peripheral circulatory problems, painful varicose veins, inflamed veins, superficial thromboses, poorly healing wounds, insect stings, sore throats, and hoarseness
How used	If not otherwise prescribed, wet compresses soaked in diluted arnica tincture (1 tablespoonful of the tincture mixed in 1 quart of water) for external application to the skin. For gargling, 10-20 drops of the tincture mixed in a glass of water.	If not otherwise prescribed, dilute 1 part of arnica tincture to 5 parts (or as much as 10 parts) of 45% alcohol or of water. Use as wet compresses or as liniment several times a day. For gargling, 1 teaspoonful of the tincture diluted in 1 glass of warm water

Note: both laboratories stress "for external use only," which includes gargling, but not swallowing. In sections 4 through 12 of this book, however, you'll see that herbal tea manufacturers occasionally include arnica in their teas. These reputable laboratories have used only the safe and properly prepared forms of arnica.

A delicious vegetable that became more than a gourmet's delight for gallbladder sufferers

Long before today's scientists succeeded in putting a finger on cynarin as the amazingly effective ingredient of the artichoke, this culinary delight already enjoyed a respectable history of relieving the distress of liver and gallbladder sufferers.

The leaves and roots of the artichoke (*Cynara scolymus*)—a tall, thistle-like vegetable most often recognized by its fist-sized, fleshy, edible flower head—are a rich source of enzymes and vitamin A, and even some vitamin B. Other ingredients stimulate the body's natural production and flow of bile, reinforce the liver's power to neutralize poisons that enter the body, promote the flow of urine, and lower the amount of sugar in the blood. It is also likely that artichoke reduces the amount of free cholesterol in the body.

Artichoke is used in gallbladder and digestion remedies recommended for people who suffer from arteriosclerosis, for people whose liver function needs bolstering after fat-rich meals, and for those who have infectious hepatitis, certain skin conditions, or excess albumin in the urine, or who need a diuretic to increase their urinary flow.

Don't confuse the above artichoke (*Cynara scolymus*) with the Jerusalem artichoke or topinambur, which is the tuber of *Helianthus tuberosus*, a food once eaten by the American Indians.

A nutrient-rich antimicrobial and anti-cancer vegetable-fruit for salads

Excavation of ancient tombs in Mexico revealed that the cultivation of avocados or alligator pears (*Persea americana*) began as long as 7000 to 8000 years ago. Only one out of every 5,000 or so blossoms on the avocado tree develops into an avocado fruit, which is sometimes thought to be a vegetable because of its beautifully textured and shiny green skin, and because of its use in salads. The delicate, nutty flavor of the pulp can be enjoyed simply with a little lime or lemon juice. Or the avocado can be mashed into a Mexican *guacamole* purée, along with cheese, onions, pepper or chillies, vinegar, and olive oil.

The nutritious avocado contains starch, protein, nutritive oils, lecithin, vitamins (A, B, C ,D ,E) and minerals. It also contains proanthocyanidine, a substance active against sarcoma—a cancerous growth. Avocado has an antimicrobial effect, is used in Asia to alleviate ulcers and colic, and is an effective ingredient of soothing and nourishing skin creams.

A group of scientists at the United States Citrus and Subtropical Products Laboratory at Winter Haven, Florida, reported that some varieties of avocado had more D-mannoheptulose than other varieties, and that this substance inhibits insulin secretion in animals, thus producing "instant diabetes" if ingested in sufficient amounts. But this should not be of any great concern because, they reported, we don't eat enough avocados to significantly affect the amount of sugar in our blood. There are indeed other foods we eat which would hurt us more if we overate them. Also, these scientists prefaced their findings with the remark that the chemical analysis of D-mannoheptulose is difficult, so perhaps their study needs further work before the effect, if any, of avocados on people predisposed to diabetes is known, they reported.

And yet, concerning avocados for diabetics, a native Haitian herbalist (who was also a European-trained pharmacist) recommended that diabetics eat a large spoonful of violet or purple avocado (the part that touches the inside of the avocado's skin) before breakfast, drink 3 cups of avocado leaf tea morning, noon and night, and also take a lot of brewer's yeast.

How outdoor people ease bites and stings with the dropsy plant

One of lemon balm (*Melissa officinalis*) or melissa's German names, *Herzkraut* or heart herb, reveals its use in quietening nervous pounding of the heart. Lemon balm's sedative effect— either from a bath or tea—supports normal heart function, particularly in excessively nervous people. Tea made from its leaves aids digestion, especially biliary function, and helps prevent gas. The tea also helps control fever, dispel migraine headache and, when used externally in wet dressings, helps mend poorly healing wounds. Outdoorsmen (and women) have relieved insect bites and stings by applying crushed lemon balm leaves to the affected spots. These effects are due to the plant's ethereal oils, tannins, bitters, mucilage, and enzymes. Lemon balm or melissa is used in quite a few of the combination remedies described later in this book.

How a rancher alleviated sore gums with a protozoan-killing berry plant

The barberry, pepperidge, piprage or jaundice berry shrub (*Berberis vulgaris*) produces edible vitamin-C-rich berries, roots from which American pioneers extracted a yellow dye, and a root bark and stems from which cardiovascular, antiparasitic and bile-promoting effects were obtained.

The *berberis* in barberry's scientific name came to Europe along with the Arabs from the Berber areas of North Africa when they conquered Spain hundreds of years ago. So, this may account for the similar-sounding *barberry* ... like the old Barbary Coast of sailing-ship days.

Barberry extracts act favorably on the heart and circulation; the plant's root bark contains substances that widen blood vessels and lower blood pressure. Barberry extracts can actually cure cutaneous leishmaniasis (a tropical disease which also goes by the names Aleppo boil, Delhi sore, oriental sore, and tropical ulcer) by inhibiting the growth of the leishmania protozoa (one-celled organisms) which cause it. The barberry has also been useful in the treatment of jaundice, gallstones and various liver ailments, as well as for fighting fevers. A Montana rancher told me that fresh ripe berry juice alleviated his pyorrhea when he chewed the berries and squished the juice through the openings between his teeth so it could get at his inflamed and painful gums. Barberry owes these effects to its alkaloids (especially barberine), tannins, fruit acids ethereal oil, polysaccharides, and other ingredients.

A legume with surprising effects for a gouty farmer and a diabetic teacher

The effects of beans (*Phaseolus vulgaris*) recently surprised some scientists, but hardly surprised some of the older folks in rural villages here and there in the world who knew all along that bean skins can decrease blood pressure as well as help control kidney disease and diabetes. Recent research at the Howard Hughes Medical Institute in Miami, Florida, indicated that there is indeed a substance in beans that blocks the body's use of starch by inhibiting the action of an enzyme involved in changing starch to glucose. This is a fact of great interest not only to obese people, but also to diabetics, whose metabolism may not be able to deal with too much glucose.

The water in which beans have been boiled is a home remedy for gout, rheumatism, kidney and bladder ailments, diabetes, and edema. Cooking destroys the toxin phasin in beans (which could cause inconveniences such as diarrhea and nausea) and makes beans palatable as well as nutritious for the many peoples in the world for whom they form one of the staple foods of life. Beans (that is, the seeds without their skins) also contain starch and protein. The skins contain amino acids, small amounts of prussic acid, silicon compounds, calcium, phosphorus, vitamin C, and other substances, including vegetable insulin or glycokinin.

For combatting gout (by reducing uric acid formation and deposition in his system), a Westphalian farmer drank the water in which his wife boiled dried bean skins. One of the village school teachers drank bean skin tea made by boiling 1 tablespoonful of dried bean skins in 1 pint of water until only ½ a pint of water remained) to help control her mild diabetes.

How a bear food alleviated urinary tract distress

The bearberry (*Arctostaphylos uva-ursi*) is a trailing evergreen shrub also known as bear's grape and kinnikinic. The *bear* part of the name is because bears—who wake up "as hungry as a bear" after their winter sleep—eagerly nibble on the berries. *Kinnikinic* is an American Indian name for a mixture of this plant with others they once used as a smoking blend. American frontiersmen did the same; they crushed handfuls of air-dried young bearberry leaves into powder, which they then smoked or chewed like tobacco. Pioneer women were well aware of bearberry's definite effect on the urinary system, and they accordingly brewed bearberry leaves into an antiseptic, astringent tea for "cleansing the kidneys," as they used to say, to clear up kidney and bladder infections such as cystitis, pyelitis, and urethritis. But the urine has to be alkaline for bearberry to act antiseptically or bactericidally.

I met an old country veterinarian in rural New York State (in plain sight of Cornell University's scientifically modern agricultural laboratories) who successfully cleared up his cows' mastitis (inflammation of the udder) by giving them bearberry tea for several days. For his own wife's cystitis, the vet boiled 2 tablespoonsful of bearberry leaves in 3 cupsful of water until only 2 cupsful of water remained in the pot ‐but *not* longer, because that would thicken the tea and make it too slimy. His wife drank only 1 pint throughout the day; she once tried to drink more of the tea, but it nauseated her. The single pint, however, relieved her condition.

Bearberry contains the phenolglycoside arbutin, tannins (too much of which can irritate overly sensitive stomachs), flavonoids, and other substances, all of which contribute to the plant's effectiveness.

A vitamin-C rich berry plant that stopped a mountain climber's diarrhea and a New Zealand woman's sore eyes

Blackberries (*Rubus fructicosus*) and raspberries (*Rubus idaeus*) are so closely related that blackberries are sometimes called black raspberries. Raspberry leaves—which are rich in vitamin C, and also contain tannins, flavonoids, and fruit acids—once held a reputation as an aphrodisiac to spark up a tired sex life. Raspberry juice or tea is a well-known thirst-quencher during bouts of fever. In England, raspberry leaf has been recommended for easing delivery of babies. A New Zealand woman told me she soothed conjunctivitis with a raspberry leaf tea eyewash.

The tannins in blackberry root (which is collected in late winter and early spring) and especially in the leaves (young ones are collected in the summer) act astringently, and thus control diarrhea and dysentery. During a long hike, I watched a mountaineer chew up fresh green blackberry leaves, sometimes on his lunch bread, to halt diarrhea. This astringent property, along with its vitamin C, is what makes gargling with root or leaf tea so helpful in alleviating tonsilitis and sore threat. Blackberry leaf mouthwash has often helped relieve inflamed gums, too.

A strongly brewed blackberry leaf tea is used for the above purposes as well as to reduce menstrual flow. Dilute leaf tea, not strong enough to make you pucker up, makes a fine breakfast beverage to replace black tea, and it is often included in breakfast tea and spring tonic tea mixes.

To prepare a store of blackberry tea leaves, collect young leaves during the plant's flowering season, dry them one day in the sun, then spread them out inside or in the shade until drying is complete. Discard any leaves that look different than the others, such as the ones on which any fungus might be growing.

Vitamin-C rich gout berries

Black currants (*Ribes nigrum*) are rich in vitamin C and also contain vitamins of the B complex and vitamin J or the anti-pneumonia factor, as well as fruit acids and pectin. The leaves contain ethereal oil, tannin, vitamin C, and rutin. Leaf tea is for kidney ailments, gout, rheumatism, throat inflammations, and convulsive coughing. Crushed fresh leaves have been rubbed on minor skin wounds to soothe and hasten healing. Black currant juice is used for kidney ailments, colicky pains, and fighting colds. Sore throats and mouths as well as bleeding gums have been eased by gargling and rinsing the mouth with dried currant tea (made by pouring a cupful of boiling water over 1 to 2 teaspoonsful of crushed dried currants). The leaf tea is brewed by pouring a cupful of boiling water over a pinch of dried leaves without the stems, and steeping 5 to 10 minutes as usual.

How a plumber helped control his diabetes
with a plant that also provides vitamin A
for good night vision, controls diarrhea,
but can loosen up constipation, too

Land is occasionally set on fire to encourage the subsequent springing up of blueberry (*Vaccinium myrtillus*) bushes (also called huckleberry, whortleberry and bilberry), thus creating a marketable crop of fruit as well as attracting blueberry-eating game for hunters—many of whom take full advantage of the blueberries, too, when living afield on hunting and camping trips. The hunters can well appreciate the diarrhea-stopping effect of the dried berries, and the night-vision-enhancing powers of the fresh fruit. Blueberries' content of vitamins of the B complex, vitamin C, and protovitamin A are part of the reason why blueberries improve night vision and even help restore vision after eye problems, as well as enhance the tone of the tiniest of the blood vessels, the capillaries.

The pectin of dried blueberries helps clear up diarrhea, especially in people with chronic gastrointestinal upsets. Fresh berries, on the other hand, can act as a laxative for some people. The berries' tannic and fruit acids act antibacterially, help clear up intestinal infections like dysentery and typhoid fever, and also help clear up eczema (see the section in this book on cleansing the blood and spring cures). Fresh blueberry juice and even jams have been used to obtain some of the above benefits.

Blueberry leaves (which contain flavoglycosides and tannins) and fruit tea gargles soothe and help to heal inflamed mucous membranes of the mouth and throat. Blueberry fruit tea can be made by boiling 1 tablespoonful of dried berries for 10 minutes in 1 cupful of water. Blueberry leaf tea, which acts as a disinfectant along the urinary tract, can be brewed in the usual way, using leaves best gathered just before the blueberries ripen.

Blueberry leaves have been brewed by diabetics, especially elderly diabetics with mild diabetes, to lower the amount of sugar in their blood. Blueberry leaf tea, however, like certain other effective herbal remedies, shouldn't be taken uninterruptedly over long periods. Alternate herbal teas throughout the year for best results.

A Berlin plumber drank an unsweetened cup of the following tea before breakfast to help control his mild diabetes, which he said bothered him much less than when he didn't drink it (and that was regardless of whether he forgot to take his other prescribed medication or not—I say *other* because his physician prescribed this tea as well as another diabetic medication): 1 tablespoon of a mixture of blueberry leaves and bean skins boiled 1 minute in a cup of water, then steeped 5 minutes.

How Chilean leaves relieved gallstone pain

Boldo (*Peumus boldus*), an evergreen shrub or small tree that grows on the dry, sun-drenched hillsides of Chile, serves as a food spice and as a medicine. The flavonoids, alkaloids, ethereal oil, and other compounds in boldo leaves account for their use in alleviating cramping, stimulating the secretion and flow of bile, improving liver and kidney function, and providing sedative and heart-toning action. That's a lot of benefit which translates specifically into alleviation of cystitis, liver pain, gallbladder pain, and the kinds of rheumatism which benefit from diuretics.

A pharmacist in Cologne relieved his gallstone distress by drinking boldo tea 3 times a day. He poured 3 cupsful of boiling water over 3 teaspoonsful of dried boldo leaves, steeped it about 5 minutes, and drank a cup of it in the morning, one at noon, and one in the evening to relieve his pain, which usually abated within several hours, or else didn't start up as badly as when he didn't drink the boldo tea.

An anti-venom plant that protects the heart

Sheep herders know from experience that sheep which graze on broom (*Sarothamnus scoparius*) seem to resist snake venom after being bitten out on the range. Laboratory tests have verified this anti-venom effect of broom. In people, broom inhibits over-excitability of the heart's conduction system, improves return of the venous blood to the heart, slows down the relaxation phase of the heartbeat cycle, and promotes good circulation in general. Alkaloids, bitters, tannins, ethereal oil, flavonoids, and other natural compounds in broom flowers, foliage, roots, and seeds contribute to these effects.

Broom, by the way, was the emblem of the Norman sovereigns of England descended from Geoffrey the Handsome, who wore the common broom plant, then called the *planta genista*, in his helmet. Thus the historians, who are always happy to find a convenient way to name some of the overwhelming number of facts in history, named Geoffrey's line of descent the *plantagenets*.

How a clover leaf improved bile production and digestion

The name *buckbean* (*Menyanthes trifoliata*) comes to us from the old Flemish *bocx boonen*, meaning goats' beans. Three of buckbean's other English common names somewhat describe the plant and its preferred soil: *bog bean, water shamrock,* and *marsh trefoil.* Three of buckbean's German names tell us immediately about the plant's use: *Magenklee* (stomach clover), *Gallkraut* (bile herb) and *Fieberklee* (fever clover). And, in fact, buckbean promotes the secretion of digestive juices, cools down fevers, and alleviates rheumatism and neuralgia. In matters of taste and of the palate, buckbean has been used to replace hops in beer, and is now used to make Boonekamp, a German schnaps... which my friend Dr. van P. keeps in his medicine chest along with angelica-containing Chartreuse and gentian schnaps!

The substances in buckbean which contribute to its effects include bitters, an alkaloid, tannin, pectin, saponin, ethereal oil, enzymes, flavonoids (including rutin), and inulin. Fructose-containing inulin, by the way, is used to bake bread for diabetics, who can easily metabolize the fructose in it.

To encourage his production of bile, a Czechoslovakian pharmacist poured 1 cupful of boiling water over 2 teaspoonsful of crushed dried buckbean leaves and steeped it for 10 to 15 minutes. Then he took sips of it, unsweetened, throughout the day. Sometimes he drank a tea he made by pouring a cupful of boiling water over 1 tablespoonful of a mixture of buckbean leaves plus wormwood leaves and flowering tops plus juniper berries plus centaury foliage, which he steeped 10 minutes before straining out the plant parts.

A tree bark that loosens up lazy bowels

The common or purging buckthorn (*Rhamnus cathartica*) is somewhat of a stronger laxative than the alder or black buckthorn (*Frangula alnus* or *Rhamnus frangula*), which is rather mild and is used especially for relieving chronic or habitual constipation and for preventing colicky cramps. California buckthorn or cascara sagrada (*Rhamnus purshiana*) is another well used laxative.

Substances in these trees which contribute to their effects include anthraglycosides like anthraquinones or emodin compounds, tannins, saponin, prussic acid glycoside, flavonoids (including rutin), bitters, pigment, and phenolglycosides.

For constipation (and the palpitations, headache, dizziness, and feeling of fullness sometimes associated with constipation), a night watchman in a paper mill drank a tea he made by briefly boiling 1 teaspoonful of *stored* bark, then steeping the tea 10 minutes before straining out the bark fragments and drinking the tea. The watchman was careful to use only the dried bark (seasoned for at least 1 year, preferably 2 years), otherwise the bark has a tendency to nauseate and gripe.

Another way to prepare well seasoned buckthorn bark as a tea is to soak 1 teaspoonful of the dried (and seasoned for at least 1 year) bark in 1 cup of cold water for about 8 hours. Constipated people have found that 1 cup of the tea in the evening is ample, and expectant mothers should not drink more than that amount.

How an aromatic reed breaks the smoking habit, aids digestion, and relieves chronic diarrhea and asthma .

Calamus—also called sweet flag, German ginger, and wild iris—has two scientific names which aptly describe the plant: *Calamus aromaticus* and *Acorus calamus. Calamus* is Latin for *reed,* and *acorus* is from Greek *akoris* for *aromatic plant* ... names which describe calamus' spicy or peppery aromatic reed-like stalks growing along the water's edge.

Smokers who wish to break the tobacco habit can chew on dried calamus rhizome chips (a rhizome is a root-like underground stem), for it has the peculiarity of mildly nauseating some smokers.

Calamus as a mouthwash relieves bad breath and stomatitis, and as a gargle soothes tissues inflamed by laryngitis. For gargling and rinsing the mouth, soak 1 teaspoonful of finely chopped rhizome in 1 cupful of cold water for 3 hours or longer, then bring it a boil and simmer for several minutes before straining.

As a tea, prepared just like the gargle and the mouthwash described above, calamus relieves indigestion, over-acidity, gastric ulcers, gas and cramping, diarrhea, as well as distress caused by liver, spleen, and gallbladder problems.

For calamus tea as a remedy for chronic diarrhea and for asthma, an Indian pharmacist from Calcutta steeped 1 ounce of powdered

calamus rhizome chips in 20 ounces of pure water for 15 minutes in
a closed porcelain bowl, strained it and used it within 24 hours so it
didn't lose its strength.

In parts of the Arabic world, calamus has been taken to stimulate
sexual activity.

Calamus is also added to bathwater to alleviate exhaustion and
nervousness, to help heal poorly healing wounds and sores, and,
generally, to stimulate sluggish metabolism. For a bath, boil 100
grams of finely chopped rhizome for 10 minutes in 1 quart of water.
Strain it and then add it to the bathwater. Bathe 2 or 3 times a week
for about a quarter of an hour each time, just as the pharmacist of
Calcutta did after a long, hot day compounding prescriptions amid
the nerve-wracking din of the bazaar where he kept shop in that busy
city.

Substances in calamus that account for these properties include
bitters, ethereal oils, resinous materials, tannins, mucilage, starch,
saponin, and vitamin C. If the soft, aromatic rhizome chips aren't
too spicy for your taste, you can simply chew on some to obtain the
benefits of some of these ingredients in calamus.

How a girl scout leader, a British businessman, and a medical student used a tiny flower to combat inflammation, cramps, and hemorrhoids

Camomile (*Matricaria chamomilla*) is known mainly for its easing
of painful menstruation and for its cramp-relieving effect, so long
taken advantage of by generations of women. The *matricaria* part of
its scientific name, in fact, comes from the Latin word *matrix* for
womb.

Camomile combats inflammation, especially of the mucous
membranes along the respiratory passages. Camomile mouthwash
soothes sore gums. Its anti-inflammatory and cramp-easing qualities
led to its use for bronchial asthma in children. Camomile promotes
healing of poorly closing wounds and of hemorrhoids. It calms down
the nerves. It relieves cramping of the digestive organs, including
the gallbladder, alleviates gas, and controls diarrhea. Camomile also
promotes sweating in ailing people who need it, but not usually in

people who don't need a good sweating out of some sickness. Camomile's ethereal oils, bitters, flavonoids, and coumarin compounds, among others, make camomile one of those "cure-all" plants that really seems to do just that   .

A girl scout leader in England eased her colpitis by douching with a quart of warm infusion prepared by pouring 1 quart of boiling water over 2 to 4 teaspoonsful of camomile flowers and steeping it for 5 minutes, and then straining it before use. This girl scout leader's teenage daughter used a camomile rinse to lighten her blondish hair!

The most, how shall I put it, "emergency" use I ever saw being made of camomile was by an older (that is, old enough to have hemorrhoids) room-mate of mine who was in my anatomy class at the University of Heidelberg. He had just returned from a five-day Volkswagen jaunt over hills and dales, and his rectal varicose veins (that's what hemorrhoids are) were quite "angry." So my room-mate layered the bottom of an enameled bucket with camomile flowers, poured 2 quarts of boiling water over them, then promptly sat right down on top of the bucket, wrapping a sheet around himself so that all the vapors bathed his hemorrhoids. This seemed to relieve his acute distress. After the "tea" cooled down a bit, he poured it into a shallow basin and sat in it—like a *sitz* bath. I have rarely seen anyone more relieved.

Here's a nasal douche which can also be used for wet dressings (gauze pads or cotton pledgets) to ease sores in the nose: pour 1 cup of boiling water over 1 teaspoonful of camomile flowers, steep 5 to 10 minutes, then use warm.

A British businessman who lived in Bombay, India, prepared his all-purpose remedy, camomile tea, freshly on the same day he planned to use it by covering 1 ounce (about 30 grams) of bruised camomile flowers with 20 ounces of boiling water and steeped it 15 minutes in a closed jar. His method was hardly different from the European way, except he steeped it somewhat longer than most Europeans do. This Bombay businessman and his fellow Britishers there brewed this tea as their one-plant medicine chest for use as wet compresses and rinses, and also as an actual tea drunk from very British tea cups. Here is a list of some of these uses:

For compresses and rinses
  Boils
  Burns
  Eyewash for irritated, inflammed or infected eyes
  Inflamed skin
  Itches

For tea
  Bladder cramps
  Bronchitis
  Colds
  Diarrhea
  Fevers
  Gallbladder problems
  Gas and flatulence
  Indigestion
  Kidney cramps
  Ulcers (gastrointestinal)
  Women's menstrual cramping

Note that camomile (sometimes spelled chamomile) with the scientific name *Matricaria chamomilla* is the standard or "real" camomile, which is also called *German* or *Hungarian* camomile to differentiate it from *Roman* camomile (scientific name *Anthemis nobilis*). Although this other, Roman, camomile is quite a different genus and species of plant, it can be used with or instead of the "real" camomile. The Roman is, however, somewhat weaker in its effects.

Camomile has a definite place in many combination herbal remedies prepared today in Europe, where serious pharmacists, physicians and other citizens expect and get safe and economical results from them.

A spice that allays colicky pains and after-dinner gas

Caraway (*Carum carvi*) "seeds" (really a seed-like fruit) aid digestion and relieve or prevent colicky pains and gas associated with the eating of certain foods. The ethereal oil in caraway seeds accounts for these gastrointestinal effects as well as for its lactation-promoting effect in nursing mothers. Caraway oil also finds good use externally in liniments to alleviate the pains of rheumatism and pleurisy (inflammation of the membranous sacs that enclose the lungs). Europeans have long enjoyed caraway not only in rye bread, but also in *Kümmel*, an excellent after-dinner liqueur that does wonders for digestion along with providing for a warm, cheery after-dinner atmosphere.

A tiny pinch of a powder composed of crushed caraway plus crushed fennel plus crushed aniseed after meals helps digestion and prevents gas; it usually relieves gas after the mixture is washed down and before its taste leaves the mouth. People who needed to "start their mouths watering" have chewed caraway seeds to encourage salivation, thus aiding good digestion.

In the Arab world, crushed fresh caraway root is applied externally to inflamed and swollen lymph nodes to lessen discomfort. A North African customs official ground up caraway seed with copper sulfate (an astringent) then mixed it with beef bone marrow to make a healing ointment for easing his hemorrhoids; he claimed they began "drawing together" right away, feeling much better in an hour or so.

A spice that eases heartburn

Cardamom or cardamon (*Elettaria cardamomum*) owes its name to the Greek word *kardia* for heart, plus *amomos* for spice because it was and still is taken for indigestion and "heartburn" (which is caused by an overly acidic digestive tract, among other things, not a burning heart). With some stretch of the imagination, the cardamom seed looks like a heart, and so this, too, may be another reason for the *kardia* in this spice's name. The flavor of curries, baked goods, and liqueurs are sparked by cardamom, particularly its ethereal oil (which is responsible for the effect on digestion).

If you brew a tea from whole cardamon "seed" (really the pods), then break the pods open and crush the tiny seeds in them for a faster brewing. A cup of tea brewed from several pinches of cardamom usually alleviates indigestion by the time the whole cupful is drunk.

A weather-predicting thistle that helped
prevent scars and heal wounds

One of the carline thistle's (*Carlina acaulis*) Alpine names is *Wetterdistel* or *weather thistle* because you can use it like a hygrometer to measure humidity: in fine, dry weather the silvery petals stay open, but they close up as wet weather threatens to approach. The root has been used to encourage sweating and the flow of urine, to promote regular menses, to improve digestion, to fight fevers, and as a worm remedy. All these properties are due to the plant's ethereal oil, tannin, inulin, resin, an enzyme, and other substances.

A Munich pharmacist used 1 teaspoonful of chopped carline thistle rootstock (but only imported ones, for the wild-growing German ones are protected by conservation law) to boil several minutes and apply as wet compresses to skin conditions and wounds; he said it helped prevent bad scars. That same pharmacist used the dried out above-ground parts of this large, round-faced, silvery, stemless flower as a holiday table centerpiece.

A poppy relative that relieved a beekeeper's
cramps

Extracts of the greater celandine or rock poppy (*Chelidonium majus*), member of the poppy family (with effects similar in some ways to those of morphine, which comes from the opium poppy, a relative of celandine) relax the nervous system; alleviate cramping in the bronchial tubes, gallbladder, and other parts of the digestive tract; and widen the coronary blood vessels, thus helping to relieve or prevent angina pectoris. Celandine also helps rid the body of uric acid, it seems, and thus helps against gout. Like papaya, celandine contains an enzyme that breaks down proteins, and this may be the reason for its use to remove warts. Herbalists recommend, however, that the sap be diluted with water or vinegar before getting it on the skin. Don't swallow it, either. Besides the enzymes, saponins, and flavonoids in celandine, its alkaloids (including berberine, also found in goldenseal and barberry, among other places in the vegetable world) are particularly responsible for many of the plant's effects, including its use to relieve cancer pain. (Such use, however, and most especially of the fresh plant, is *not* for the inexperienced. Consult an herbally qualified physician for guidance.) A central European beekeeper said he derived some of this plant's uncramping benefits by pouring a cupful of boiling water over 1 to 2 teaspoonsful of the dried root or foliage for the tea he drank between meals for several weeks.

How a doctor from India overcame gas and sleeplessness

Celery (*Apium graveolens*) promotes the flow of urine, alleviates gas and heartburn, and eases nervous restlessness as well as rheumatism, gout, and rheumatoid arthritis, especially in people who also suffer from mental depression. Remedies may include extracts of celery root and celery "seed" (really a seed-like fruit) as well as the stalks and leaves, these various parts containing ethereal oil, flavonoids, bitters, inositol (a vitamin-like nutrient), thiamine, vitamin C, potassium, asparagine, choline, and other natural compounds.

Dandelion seems to reinforce the beneficial effects of celery, and these two plants have been combined by some suffers in the same tea for alleviating their rheumatic distress.

An Indian doctor from New Delhi boiled 4 ounces of coarsely crumbled celery seed in 40 ounces of water in a pyrex fireproof glass bowl until only 20 ounces of water was left. He strained the plant parts out and discarded them, leaving the tea, of which he took 1/4 to 1 ounce to combat gas and to calm him down enough to fall asleep much sooner that the hour or so it usually took when insomnia was troubling him. For his wife's nervousness and rheumatism, he combined the celery tea with buckbean leaf tea.

Celery *seed* is no stranger to American kitchens, celery *soda* used to be seen in delicatessens years ago much more frequently than now, and celery *root* is still in everyday European use for soups and salads. (An Italian cook near Chicago often shredded the large, turnip-like root of celeriac—*Apium graveolens rapaceum*—in his salads.) So celery stalks and foliage are only part of the celery story

A bitter herb that aids digestion and relieves skin conditions by cleansing the blood under it

Centaury (*Gentiana centaurium* or *Chironia centaurium*) is a bitter tonic herb with essentially the same digestion-stimulating effects as gentian, hence the *Gentiana* part of its scientific name. *Chironia*, part of another of the plant's names, alludes to Chiron the *centaury* or mythical half-man and half horse—medical teacher of Achilles and Asclepius. Chiron is said to have discovered the curative properties of this plant, which contains bitters, flavonoids, saponin, etc.

A Swiss apothecary gave his family members 2 cups of centaury tea daily (prepared by soaking 2 teaspoonsful of crushed foliage in 2 cupfuls of cold water overnight, or else pouring boiling water over the foliage and steeping it for 10 minutes before straining out the plant parts) for heartburn, liver and gallbladder function, gout, skin conditions, and to cleanse the blood (thus contributing to skin health from the inside out, which is what blood "cleansers" and "purifiers" really do, among other things).

Two other scientific names for centaury, in case you try to look them up somewhere, are *Erythraea centaurium* and *Centaurium minus*.

A coffee-like root that eased bloodshot eyes and gallbladder problems

Chicory or succory (*Cichorium intybus*) is a humble yet attractive flowering plant that grows modestly along the edges of fields and roadways, hence its German name *Wegwarte*—one who waits by or keeps watch on the roads. Chicory's tatter-ended blue flowers are aptly named *blue* or *ragged sailors*, as well as *blue daisy* and *blue dandelion*.

Extract of chicory root widens the blood vessels. Leaf extract, however, narrows them (in experiments on animals), but does favorably affect our stomach and gallbladder functions, especially when the chicory extract is combined with an extract of bitter orange. Such effects are due to the chicory's tannin, bitters, coumarin, and inulin, among other substances, and the substances in the bitter orange when it's used combined with chicory.

Chicory leaves and sprouts (*witloof* to the Belgians) go nicely into salads, and the root makes a coffee substitute when roasted, which converts some of the compounds in the root into caramel, and develops a coffee-like aroma. Belgians and other coffee-lovers often add chicory root to coffee for enhancing flavor and aroma. (*Witloof* or the chicory spear, sometimes called endive, is a Belgian national vegetable.) The following remedy is from my 1975 winter and spring notebook that I filled during my stay in a village near Turnhout in the north of Belgium, just near the Dutch border:

A Belgian pharmacist suggested boiling 2 to 4 grams of chopped chicory root, leaves or flowers in a cup of water for 3 minutes, dipping a gauze pad or cotton pledget into it, and applying it to inflamed and bloodshot eyes for almost immediate relief. I tried it the morning after I sat with him all night in a cigar-smoked filled taproom, where we sort of scientifically tested several bottles of good stiff herbal schnaps ... all of which, of course, irritated our eyes quite a bit. The cool chicory eyewash did help within minutes.

When my Belgian cousin's gall bladder and digestion didn't work better after a cup of Belgian coffee mixed with chicory, then he drank plain chicory root tea made by pouring 2 cupsful of boiling water over 1 teaspoonful of ground chicory root, and steeping it for 10 minutes before straining out the grounds. This tea usually helped his digestion quite rapidly.

Because cornflowers or bluebottle flowers (*Centaurea cyanus*) contain bitters and the same glycoside (cichorin) found in chicory, their extract is often used for the same digestion-promoting effects as those obtained with chicory.

Pure, concentrated aromatic oils from drugstores and gourmet shops

The pure, distilled, concentrated aromatic oils available at your drugstore, gourmet or bake shop, or even the supermarket, have their normal, healthy use in foods, cosmetics and pharmaceutical products. They have also been used separately, dropwise or less, in helpful teas and other remedies. However, don't use too much of these oils by themselves as remedies. They can be too strong, and you don't have the leeway you have with teas and decoctions made from leaves, flowers, or other plant parts, in which very much less of active substances get loose into the water, thus giving you a milder dosage. One or two drops of the oils (but only pure, medical and/or food grade) are sufficient.

An antiseptic spice that relieves gastro-intestinal and menstrual distress

Cinnamon (*Cinnamomum ceylanicum*) is named after the Arabic *kinnamon*, which comes from *qaneh*, meaning cane or reed, which is just how cinnamon stems look. Even the sticks (the curled "quills" of inner bark that some people buy instead of powder) look like reeds.

Many so-called cinnamon-flavored foods contain more synthetic cinnamon than the genuine article, so if you want to use cinnamon for a remedy, or use any other spice for that matter, you'd do well to make sure that you have real spice.

Cinnamon generally strengthens and stimulates the stomach. Specifically, cinnamon relieves gas, enteritis, nausea, heartburn, and menstrual distress (partly by calming the nerves), as illustrated by Mary C.'s relief within a short time after—or even during—drinking a cup or so of cinnamon tea. It's strongly antiseptic, which is quite understandable when you realize that the ethereal oil in cinnamon contains eugenol, an antiseptic and pain-killing substance.

A pain-killing spice for teeth and ears

Eugenol is also in another spice—cloves (*Eugenia aromatica*, *Eugenia caryophyllus*, etc.), and clove oil you can buy for earaches and toothaches; when I chewed two clove buds for my own toothache, it seemed to work within five minutes—but you must keep the chewed-up cloves off your tongue, or it burns. Clove powder and tea are dispensed by pharmacists in India, where cloves are recognized as a stimulating aromatic spice with the power to combat gas, nausea, and vomiting. An Algerian teacher told me she drank clove tea to control nausea and diarrhea, one cupful of tea brewed from a large pinch of crushed cloves—but she added that there are better remedies for diarrhea. Clove oil is obtainable at many drugstores as an earache and toothache remedy

A family of stimulating, calming, anti-cramping, and vitamin C-rich fruits

Citrus fruits, as everyone knows, are oranges, lemons, limes, and grapefruit. Unfortunately, however, it is not so simple to say orange, for example, and have everyone know just what *kind* of orange is meant. Does *orange* mean *sweet* orange, *Seville* (or bitter or sour) orange, or *Bergamot* orange? Curative and other properties may differ from one kind of orange to the other. Then there are lemons, limes, citrons, shaddocks, and so on.

In general, citrus fruit juices and oils are often used to sweeten remedies containing other plants or to mask unpleasant tastes in such remedies. Some citrus fruit does, however, exert certain effects. One wonders whether orange blossoms are used at weddings because of their stimulating effects (which you could obtain if you brewed the dried blossoms into a tea) or because of their hypnotic effects (obtained by inhaling their distilled oils)! Seville orange blossoms provide ethereal oils used in perfumery—and perfumes can certainly stimulate the physiology and psychology of persons exposed to them. Those oils can also relieve digestive and bronchial cramping. Sweet orange rind (containing ethereal oils, flavonoids, bitters, alkaloids, etc) and leaves stimulate the flow of digestive juices and prevent gas. The People's Republic of China currently uses oranges to combat inflammations, infections, and diarrhea; to lower blood pressure; to improve gallbladder function; and to calm down overactive response and hyperexcitability, including convulsions and epilepsy.

Lemon rind is aromatic and bitter, so it aids digestion. Lemon juice stops indigestion, cools down fevers, and clears up as well as prevents scurvy. Lime does the same: it was lime juice that finally let Britain's sailors overcome the scourge of scurvy on long sea voyages, hence their nickname "limey "

Although citrus fruits offer large amounts of vitamin C, there are other plants described in this book which contain much more of that vitamin.

An antibacterial, resistance-building, immunity-stimulating root that also kills insects

Narrow-leaved purple coneflower or black Sampson (*Echinacea angustifolia*) root grows on prairies and dry sandy areas in the United States. The bacteria-inhibiting and cortisone-like substances extracted from it contribute to this plant's power to help clear up infections (including boils and abscesses) and to promote the healing of wounds by supporting the body's own natural resistance, and by stepping up the tissue's regenerative powers. Coneflower stimulates the lymphatic system, which is involved with immunity and antibodies that protect us against harmful substances that invade the body. Coneflower, in addition, also contains a substance with insecticidal powers (but only on insects, so it won't affect us).

A pain-relieving, sleep-inducing yellow flower that eased a barber's bronchitis, arthritis and rheumatism

Wine made from cowslip or primrose (*Primula veris, Primula officinalis*) flowers allays pain and brings on sleep. The saponins, especially in the root, make cowslip useful in clearing phlegm out of the throat and chest of bronchitis and pneumonia sufferers. The phenolglycosides, ethereal oil, silicon, tannin, flavonoids, and other substances in cowslip contribute, too, to cowslip's other effects. These include, according to a barber from Passau near the Bavarian Forest, relief of gout and rheumatism, but only if the dark-yellow and strongly scented flowers are boiled in wine. He drank a cup of it just at bedtime, keeping up this nightcap habit for months. The barber said that he suffered less attacks during these months, and the attacks which he did have were milder than when he didn't drink cowslip tea at all. That barber also made a tea for arthritis and nervous headache by pouring half a cupful of boiling water over a few teaspoonsful of dried cowslip foliage and flowers. Sometimes, too, he made a tea to get phlegm up when he had bronchitis by boiling a few teaspoonsful of chopped cowslip root in a cupful of water ·

One of our commonest weed flowers with the most surprising effects on health

Dandelion (*Taraxacum officinale*), as befits a long-known and long-used plant, has a long list of other names which include blowball, lion's tooth or *dent-de-lion* in French (from which we get the name *dandelion* in English), cankerwort, white endive, Irish daisy, and a French name which refers to dandelion's diuretic effects—*pisse-en-lit*. Dandelion's scientific name, *Taraxacum officinale*, refers to its ancient use in cases of eye inflammation (*taraxis*) + its effect (*akeomai*, I heal), and its acceptance in medicine for official use (*officinale*).

Besides promoting the flow of urine and the removal of excess water (particularly when water retention is caused by liver problems), dandelion also promotes bile secretion and acts as a spring tonic for persons suffering from chronic anemia and chronic eczema; it also reportedly stimulates heart function. Dandelion relieves rheumatism, gout, chronic indigestion, and constipation. The root extract stimulates glandular activity and increases the respiratory capability of our blood cells and tissues. Like chicory root, dandelion root can be roasted, pulverized, and brewed into a coffee-like beverage, and dandelion leaves can be tossed into an ideal spring blood-cleansing salad.

Pharmacologists and others at first thought that dandelion's vitamin C was the main reason for its curative properties, so long taken advantage of by kings and commoners alike. Research, however, verified that it was also dandelion's bitters, inositol, tannins, ethereal oil, resins, inulin, amino acids, xanthophyll (a yellow pigment discussed in the section on stinging nettle), niacin, and other substances that contribute to its healthful properties.

A British pharmacist prepared his standard dandelion tea by putting 1 to 2 teaspoonsful of chopped dandelion root and foliage in a cupful of cold water, bringing it to a boil, removing it from the heat and steeping it for 15 minutes before straining out the plant parts.

How a physician proved that a frankly astonishing non-steroid anti-rheumatic root lacked any side effects

The secondary storage roots of the devil's claw or grapple plant (*Harpagophytum procumbens*) from the drier parts of South Africa contain anti-rheumatic substances that counter rheumatic inflammation and protect against inflamed and swollen joints. This protection consists not only in symptomatic alleviation of pain, but also of actual improvement in the disrupted bodily functions that cause some of the pain. Native African herbalists also used devil's claw as a remedy against gallbladder, liver, kidney, and bladder ailments. Bitters and glycosides are among the substances that make this plant an effective remedy for so many sufferers of arthritis and rheumatism.

A West German physician tested devil's claw according to the methods used to evaluate new drugs synthesized by the pharmaceutical industry. He treated one group of 25 patients with the remedy being studied, in this case devil's claw. He also treated a similar, second group of 25 patients with a standard non-steroid anti-rheumatic drug, phenylbutazone. Then, after 28 days of treatment, he compared both groups—each of which was composed of 25 rheumatic sufferers (5 of them with gout) all of comparable age, sex and symptoms—for their reactions to the treatments. The table summarizes what the comparison showed:

	Group I (Devil's claw)	Group II (Phenylbutazone)
Total improvement (morning stiffness, pain, sleeplessness) for rheumatism	80%	72%
Side effects	None	16% (4 patients)
Total improvement for gout	80%	40%
Side effects	None	8% (2 patients)

The physician concluded from his study that devil's claw tablets (each containing 410 milligrams of extract, at a dosage of 3 tablets a day for 28 days) was at least as effective as the standard phenylbutazone for treating rheumatism and gout. (The dosage of phenylbutazone was started at 3 pills a day, but had to be reduced after 5 days because of its cumulative effect.) The most significant finding was the *lack of any side effects or intolerance* in the devil's claw group.

Surprisingly successful uses of devil's claw have been reported, too, by dozens of sufferers themselves, some of whose stories are told in *Miracle Health Secrets of the Old Country* (by Howard H. Hirschhorn, Parker Publishing Company, 1981) .

A milk-stimulating spice that allays digestive distress

Dill, long used in kitchens, figures in an old European bridal spell to be uttered by the bride under her breath just as she takes her marriage vows·

> I've got mustard and dill,
> Husband, when I talk you keep still!

Dill (*Anethum graveolens*) gets its name from old Norse *dilla*, meaning *to lull*, which it does indeed do to upset nerves and digestion. Dill tea has been used to lull babies to sleep, and, in adults, to relieve gas and griping, and alleviate headaches due to colds. Fresh dill juice is rubbed in externally to quickly relieve hemorrhoidal distress. The ethereal oil in dill's seed-like fruit and foliage accounts for its gas-relieving, cramp-easing effects (during or soon after drinking a cupful or so) which are also found in some other common kitchen spices. Its milk-promoting effect is probably one of the reasons why Indian physicians sometimes prescribe dill cordial (about 1/2 to 1 ounce) to new mothers just after their confinement. An African told me he drank dill tea and ate fresh dill to calm down his hiccoughs, but he didn't say how long it took to work.

The living pharmacy tree that lets a pain-wracked ferryman sleep comfortably

The black or sweet elder (*Sambucus nigra*) bush, once called a living pharmacy, may grow to tree size of over 20 feet. The first part of its scientific name, *Sambucus*, is the ancient Latin name of the plant as well as the name of the flute the ancients made of the straight stems, but only after poking out the toxic pith. American Indians, too, made flutes and elk-calling whistles from hollowed-out elder stems. The elder has been around long enough for quite a few early American grandmothers to have brewed many a hot cup of elder tea or elderberry wine with which to fight the ills of winter. I remember one of the very first books I had read to me as a child was about a kind family of field mice who took in poor half-frozen grasshopper green and spoon-fed him hot elderbery wine to revive him!

Elder's ethereal oil, flavonoids (like rutin), sweat-producing glycosides, sambucin (an alkaloid), prussic acid glycosides, bitters, tannins, saponins, fruit acids, vitamins A and C, are all some of the reasons that hot elderberry wine has on many a frosty evening warmed the insides of rural folks and nipped a beginning cold in the bud. Elder flowers as a hot tea actually sweat out colds and other winter ills. The raw, ripe berries are not considered toxic, although the green, unripe berries may theoretically be toxic because of the prussic acid in them. Some people have reported diarrhea and vomiting after eating the uncooked berries. Another species, the American black elder (*Sambucus canadensis*) is reported to be poisonous, although its *cooked* berries are reported to be safe, and have been safe in pies and preserves. Yet another species, red elder (*Sambucus racemosa*) has berries suitable for jams *after* the poisonous seeds are removed from them.

Berries, bark and root of the elder have long been used to clear up sore throats and mouths, allay neuralgia and rheumatic pains, loosen up constipation, promote the flow of urine, and enhance vascular function.

Twice a day for his rheumatism, a Swedish ferryman poured 1 cup of boiling water over 1 tablespoonful of elder flowers, steeped it 5 minutes, and drank it warm. This hot elder flower tea eased up his aches and pains so he could at least get into a comfortable position on his bunk bed and get some sleep when he wasn't on watch.

The Australian fever tree and the evergreens

Eucalyptus, blue gum or Australian fever tree (*Eucalyptus globulus*), is an evergreen tree, sometimes growing to a height of 300 or more feet, originally from Australia and Tasmania. The name *eucalyptus* is a compound of Greek *eu* (well or good) plus *kalyptos* (covered), referring to how the flower buds are covered and protected until they blossom.

Rome was once subjected to periodic bouts of "bad air" (*mal'aria* as the ancients said in Italian) from nearby marshes, a notorius breeding place for malaria-carrying mosquitos. The "bad air" was eventually made safer by the large-scale planting there of eucalyptus trees, which soak up a lot of water. And interestingly enough, eucalyptus as a remedy actually reduces fevers in people as well as in swamps! It also acts antiseptically in the urinary and respiratory passages, helps get phlegm and other secretions up from the chest, where the ethereal oils in eucalyptus loosen mucus by stimulating the ciliated cells along the respiratory passages to sweep more effectively with their tiny, hair-like whips, thus clearing the way for unhampered breathing. Eucalyptus liniment helps alleviate rheumatic pains. The eucalyptus tree also prevents the extinction of a cuddly marsupial, the koala bear, whose only food consists of eucalyptus leaves.

How a sawmill chemist got phlegm up with evergreens that also calm you down, overcome insomnia, relieve neuralgia, and alleviate eczema

Many kinds of evergreen trees (pines, firs and spruces of the *Pinus*, *Picea* and *Abies* species) contain ethereal oils, resins and other substances which have relieved human ailments for ages. Ask an asthma sufferer or someone with shortness of breath, or with a lung condition, how a walk in a pine forest affected him. Chances are that he felt better. Inhalation baths, liniments, teas and ointments made from pine, fir, and spruce trees can alleviate rheumatism, gout, menstrual discomfort, chest conditions with heavy secretions, and skin conditions. Extracts from evergreen needles improve peripheral circulation, that is, the part of the blood flow nearest to the skin, especially in the limbs; promote the flow of urine; dampen nervousness; and generally engender a feeling of healthful wellbeing throughout the body and mind.

Some evergreen buds, such as those from spruce, are rich in vitamin C and have been used to prevent and cure scurvy.

The phenols in pine tar distilled from pine wood are antiseptic and help rebuild broken tissues in some chronic skin conditions. The pine substances in baths can be varied so as to provide the best effects for a particular ailment: pine *needle* and *twig* baths contain ethereal oil and tannin, pine *oil* extract has no tannins but is full of ethereal oil, whereas pine *wood* has less ethereal oil and pine *bark* has more tannin.

A few words about bathing should be said here. Very hot baths put a burden on persons with weakened health. They should only take them with a physician's approval, and even then, weakened or elderly bathers should always have someone nearby. Warm, not hot, baths are milder and more judicious. Unless otherwise recommended, 15 or 20 minutes is long enough in the medicated bath. Don't forget that what you add to your bathwater often penetrates your skin and enters your system. Vapors rising from the surface of the warm water, too, let you inhale some of the substances in the water, especially if they contain ethereal oils (and that's why ethereal oils are also called *volatile* oils—they volatize or diffuse into the air rapidly). All that, of course, can be good for you. A good bath can make you feel as though you've had a good workout or a long walk. So, a short rest on your bed or sofa after an invigorating bath is advisable. Some of the other baths mentioned in this book can relax you so much that you really can become drowsy and might even start to slip down more and more into your bathwater. So when you just reach a comfortable drowsiness and relaxation, climb right into bed for a restful night's sleep.

A purple flowering plant that brightened a pharmacist's strained and bloodshot eyes

The reddish-purple or violet-and-white flowered eyebright (*Euphrasia officinalis*—not to be confused with American centaury or wild succory, which is *Sabatia angularis*, but sometimes also called eyebright)—cleanses and soothes the eyes as well as reportedly strengthens vision. A Veronese pharmacist who strained his eyes by repairing watches in his spare time, boiled up a thick mash of eyebright leaves and applied them to his overworked, bloodshot eyes for half an hour at a time, thus enjoying immediate relief. At other times, he poured boiling water (anywhere from 6 ounces to a pint) over dried foliage (anywhere from 1 teaspoonful to 1 tablespoonful), steeped 10 minutes, let it cool down to lukewarm, then soaked sterile cotton balls or gauze pads in it, then applied these to his burning, aching eyes. Or, he put the tea in an eyewash cup and held that directly up to his eyes. He also found that coltsfoot (*Tussilago farfara*) leaves, brewed as a tea, soothed his bloodshot eyes.

The pharmacist's wife, who swore by camomile tea (which often relieved her cramps), added it to eyebright whenever she had occasion to mix up her husband's eyewash for him. She poured a cupful of boiling water over 5 tablespoonsful of a half-and-half mixture of eyebright foliage and camomile flowers, steeped it 10 minutes, then applied it as hot as her husband could stand it— especially to relieve his sty—and repeated this treatment several times a day as needed.

A spice used by a doctor for gas and by pharmacists for tired eyes and lumbago

Fennel (*Foeniculum vulgare*), one of the classic culinary spices, gets it name from the Latin word for hay, *foenum*, because of the similarity in smell, at least in some cases and to some noses. Fennel grows so well on pasture lands that farmers and stockmen often consider it a nuisance. Fennel's ethereal oil improves stomach function, relieves cramping, expels gas, gets phlegm up out of the throat, promotes the flow of urine, and stimulates lactation in nursing mothers.

A Bombay physician used a fennel tea (1 pint of boiling water poured over about 10 grams of crushed fennel seed-like fruit) enema to expel gas. When, instead of using it as an enema, he drank fennel tea to relieve gas, he made it somewhat stronger (25 grams per pint of water); gas was expelled after drinking a cupful or so of the tea.

Like eyebright, fennel has often relieved eye conditions. Whenever her eyes felt tired and strained, a Strassbourg pharmacist bathed them (to strengthen them, she said) for about 20 minutes by covering them with a clean cloth soaked in fennel tea, which she made by boiling 1 to 2 teaspoonsful of crushed fennel "seed" for about 2 minutes in 1 cup of water, then steeping it 10 minutes before straining out the fennel pieces. She reported that her eyes began to feel better halfway through the treatment.

A Moroccan pharmacist soaked fennel in oil (any convenient edible oil, such as olive), then warmed it up before he rubbed it on himself as a liniment to relieve rheumatic aches and lumbago; he began to feel better by the time he had massaged the oil into his skin.

How an inventor soothed his hurt fingers with a textile plant that also moves bowels.

The word *flax* comes from the Anglo-Saxon *fleax* and *flechten*, meaning *to braid*, which was how this plant's fibers were used. In fact, flax (*Linum usitatissimum*) was used so much for so many things that the second part of its scientific name, *usitatissimum*, means *very useful*. Linen, flax's other common English name, comes from Greek *linon* and Celtic *llin*, both meaning *fiber* or *thread*, which the ancients made from this plant, known and cultivated by the Egyptians and others three thousand years ago.

The pain-relieving local anesthetic effect of linseed poultice and liniments on skin inflammations and purulent wounds is probably due to the glycoside linamarin in them, which liberates prussic acid when the seeds are crushed and ground; linseed's mucilage and oils also contribute to the soothing action.

Unbroken linseed act as a natural laxative because they simply swell up to provide bulk, thus stimulating normal intestinal movement without irritating the intestinal walls. A tablespoonful of crushed linseed alone or mixed with applesauce or water and taken about twice a day loosens up the bowels in a day or so. If your stomach is overly acidic, then it's better not to keep taking linseed for extended periods.

A British inventor who had his share of sore fingers and arms from little accidents in his workshop, relieved his inflammations and festered fingers by using linseed meal the way he learned from his mother to do it (and she learned it in New Delhi): he stirred 4 ounces of crushed linseed smoothly into 10 ounces of water just poured from a boiling kettle, then spooned the mix into a muslin bag (coated on the outside with olive oil to protect the skin), and applied the bag as hot as he could stand it over the inflamed or festered spot.

Another way to make a linseed bag is to fill a freshly boiled white sock halfway with whole linseed, soak the filled sock 4 to 6 hours in cold water until the linseeds swell up, then bring the whole soaked sock to a boil and steep it 10 to 20 minutes after you take the pot off the heat.

How a plant that promotes milk secretion in nursing mothers also reduces the amount of sugar in diabetics

Galega or goat's rue (*Galega officinalis*) has a name derived from Greek *gala* (milk) plus *agein* (to promote or secrete), thus referring to the plant's age-old use to increase lactation in nursing mothers. One of the substances, galegin, in galega is responsible for another interesting effect: reduction in the amount of sugar in the blood and urine (although it can cause a very transitory increase in blood sugar before it gets around to causing a longer-lasting drop in blood sugar). Some research has suggested that it's better for diabetics not to rely on galega tea for this purpose, unless for short periods, and always in conjunction with any prescribed diabetic medication already being taken; there are other, better anti-diabetic plants mentioned in this book. Externally, extracts of galega have been used to intensify the effects of X-rays in the treatment of skin tumors·

European diabetics have drunk (before each meal) a tea made by pouring a cupful of boiling water over a heaping teaspoonful of galega foliage. Another method used was 1 teaspoonful of foliage soaked in 1 cupful of cold water for 5 minutes, then brought to a boil, and finally removed from the heat and left to steep 10 minutes before straining out the plant parts.

A vegetable pollution filter with digestive, anti-infective, and cardiovascular properties

Long before garlic (*Allium sativa*) was shown to contain vitamins (A, B1, B2, niacin, C), enzymes and a sexual hormone-like substance, it was successfully used to promote digestion, regulate liver and gallbladder function, relieve cramps, expel gas, fight intestinal infections, help overcome respiratory infections, bring up phlegm, favorably affect the endocrine glands and, in general, help counter the toxic effects of environment on our body's systems. Garlic builds up the body's resistance to disease. Farmers and good cooks have known for centuries that garlic helps the heart and blood vessels. Now science has verified that it indeed can help control blood pressure within normal limits as well as prevent conditions associated with arteriosclerosis and hypertension, including reduction of the amount of cholesterol in the blood. Garlic has often been used as a supplement in the treatment of people suffering from chronic coronary insufficiency, and menopausal distress.

How a railroader alleviated chronic indigestion with a bitter herb that also increases the number of blood cells and relieves rheumatoid arthritis

Gentian (*Gentiana lutea*), also called yellow or pale gentian, is named after the Illyrian King Gentius, who reigned from 180 to 167 B.C., because he is said to have discovered the medicinal worth of the plant's root. Gentian bitters, like bitters in other plants such as chicory, can spark your tired appetite and improve your digestive processes. One drop of amarogentine, one of the bitter principles isolated from gentian, is so bitter that it can be tasted even when diluted with 50,000 drops of water. The last time I strained my eyes to read the tiniest of tiny print on a bottle of angostura bitters behind a bar to see if there was any angostura bark extract in it, I didn't find any, but I did find that the "angostura" bitters contained gentian. So I guess that's what helps some mixed drinks to stimulate your appetite.

Gentian extracts are believed to increase the number of red and white blood cells, thus helping convalescents overcome anemia and infections. It's the gentianine (an alkaloid reported to have an anti-inflammatory effect) in gentian root that explains why the Chinese use gentian as an anti-inflammatory drug to alleviate rheumatoid arthritis. (Interestingly, another quite bitter plant, devil's claw, also allays rheumatic and arthritic pain by reducing inflammation.)

A Belgian railroader alleviated his chronic indigestion by drinking 1 cup of gentian root tea (1 teaspoonful of root chips boiled 1 to 2 minutes and steeped 10 minutes) daily 30 minutes before his main meal of the day. For his nervous headaches, he drank this tea twice a day before meals, but that usually relieved only the headaches caused by his indigestion. An Austrian doctor whom I told about that case remarked that gentian tea wouldn't be too good for people who suffered from hyperacidic gastritis or acid stomach. Also he suggested two other dosages he knew about: (1) boil half a teaspoonful of root chips 5 minutes in 1 cupful of water, then take 1 to 2 tablespoonsful of it a day, and (2) take a small pinch of powdered gentian root before each of the day's three meals.

How the author of this book personally tested an Oriental root for improved digestion and sex, plus mental and physical rejuvenation

Ginseng root (*Panax ginseng, Panax quinquefolius, Eleuthero-coccus senticosus*) strengthens the inner organs, activates the mind, wards off nervous fatigue, and sparks up weakened powers of concentration. It's often used to aid digestion, prevent nausea, and increase sexual interest and powers. These, and many more, are the claims of many Orientals and quite a few Westerners.

Because so much has been claimed for ginseng, one tends to think it's a nostrum. But the results of overenthusiasm should not obscure any of its rightfully claimed properties. As early in our modern scientific era as October 1925, the 6th Congress of the Far Eastern Association of Tropical Medicine, meeting in Tokyo, Japan, reported that the pharmacological effects of Korean ginseng were similar to those of yohimbine—an alkaloid from *Corynanthe johimbe*—once used as an aphrodisiac and local anesthetic. And there are people who have tried ginseng and had interesting results. I am one of them. I was recently working on a botanical project in a European laboratory where chemists and pharmacists were analyzing ginseng elixir, that is, ginseng root extract prepared as a sort of liqueur wine. Because the quality control looked so good, I decided to try some. Now, I'm *not* what you'd call an old man (I'm 48 at the time of this writing) nor do I need any of ginseng's effects, but I drank several bottles of the elixir over three to four weeks' time . . . and to tell the truth, I don't know whether I or my wife was more surprised with the results. Perhaps it was all merely mind over matter, I'm still not sure.

Although ginseng is cultivated as a crop, the wild roots are highly prized, and are still hunted for, the oldest and most complete roots bringing the greatest price. Six years from sowing to harvest represents a normal growth period . . . and some venerable ginseng roots are over a hundred years old. Chinese sources inform me that the collection of wild ginseng there (where it was known as the *pearl of northern China*) involves two field teams: a search party plus a digging crew. The search party finds then tags (with a red thread) the ginseng plants, then the digging crew goes to work (often with spades made of deer antlers) to carefully remove the long, fibrous roots with as little loss of rootlets as possible.

The Chinese, according to one of their Hong Kong outlets, Teck Soon Hong Limited, recommend the following ways to enjoy taking your ginseng medicine (if you choose not to drink it as a cordial-like elixir, which I did in Germany):

1. Grind ginseng into powder and take it with boiled water.
2. Or cut the ginseng into slices and chew them until they dissolve in the mouth.

3. Usually, however, ginseng slices are stewed along with chicken, duck, and/or lean pork for 3 to 4 hours.

China is now exporting wild ginseng as well as cultivated varieties, some of them canned.

The Chinese also have another ginseng called tienchi (*Panax pseudo-ginseng*). As a wound remedy, tienchi earned the name of *mountain lacquer* because it healed gaping wounds, that is, closed them up as if they were being glued together. Not only did Japanese investigators (according to my Chinese sources) discover that "the effective ginseng components in tienchi were even greater than in ordinary ginsengs," but Chinese studies at Kunming, Peking and Wuhan hospitals showed that tienchi was effective in healing heart disease and arteriosclerosis, in lowering blood pressure, and in reducing excess cholesterol and hyperlipemia.

To cook tienchi, the Chinese recommend the following:
1. Pound the tienchi into small pieces, or else soften by heating over medium heat.
2. Slice and dry in the sun, or else fry in vegetable oil over medium heat, but avoid scorching it.
3. Pound again.
4. Add meat (chicken, pigs' feet, squab or mutton).
5. Stew for 3 to 4 hours.

The Chinese export tienchi whole or in slices for cookery, and powdered for sprinkling on wounds.

How a pharmacist eased sores and gum boils with a urine-promoting, antiseptic, anti-arthritic, tooth-tightening plant

The cossacks of a bygone era drank goldenrod (*Solidago virgaurea*) tea to ease kidney pain and incontinence ... perhaps caused by too much jouncing around on their galloping war horses. Goldenrod—which promotes urinary flow and encourages good kidney function—has been recommended for conditions on both sides of normal, that is, to relieve urine retention as well as to stop bedwetting. Goldenrod's blood cleansing properties help in cases of gouty, inflamed joints. Goldenrod has also been used for tightening up loose teeth, clearing up gum boils, acting antiseptically on bladder and other inflammations, and for mildly stimulating bronchial secretions. Saponins, bitters, flavonoids, an alkaloid-like substance, niacin, tannins, etheral oil, and other substances in goldenrod account for these effects.

An upstate New York pharmacist who crushed and rubbed fresh goldenrod leaves on bothersome sores and insect stings, made a diuretic tea (which also firmed up loose bowels) by pouring a cupful of boiling water over half a teaspoonful (or up to a whole tablespoonful) of dried flowering tops, then steeped 5 minutes before straining out the plant parts. For his gum boils, he brewed the tea somewhat stronger

The amazing grapes of health and the medical use of wine

Ripe grapes have long been known to be nutritious, promote the flow of urine, cool down fevers, and move the bowels. Grapes are a product of the vine (*Vitis vinifera*), whose scientific name *Vitis* is from Latin *vieo* (meaning *to bind*) because of the vine's numerous tendrils that hold and bind it to the trellis. The *vinifera* part of the name means vine- or wine-bearing. The English word *grape* comes from old French *grappe* (meaning a *bunch* or *cluster*), and an old Germanic word, *chrapho* (meaning *hook* or *claw*), again referring to the vine's curling tendril's. Grapes are probably responsible for one of our country's early names—Vinland. Norse sailor-warriors, the Vikings, found what looked to them like vines or vineyards growing in what was probably the future New England or even as far south as the future New Jersey, and called the place Vinland . centuries before the Italian navigator Columbus discovered America by mistake under the auspices of the Spanish crown!

The Wine Advisory Board of California made the following eight points about the healthful uses of wine (which agrees in essence with what the medieval physician and scholar Maimonides wrote while living in a Moslem culture which forbade the enjoyment of alcohol!):

1. Wine is generally indicated as a mild tranquilizing agent to counter emotional tension and anxiety.
2. Wine may be a useful component of the normal diet, providing energy and aiding digestive processes.
3. Dry (non-sweet) wine may be a useful source of energy and a valuable psychological addition to diabetic diets, since alcohol is metabolized without participation of insulin.
4. Dry wines have been used effectively to stimulate appetite for sufferers of such disorders as anorexia nervosa.
5. Presumably because of table and dessert wines' tranquilizing action, they have been helpful in maintaining obese patients on prescribed reducing diets.
6. Wine has been beneficial as a tranquilizing agent for sufferers of cardiovascular diseases. It may also be useful where there is a need for dilation of peripheral blood vessels, improving dull diets, and protecting against anginal attacks. Recent statistics suggest that wine in the diet may act as a general protective factor against coronary disease.
7. Wine may be most important in the care of convalescent and especially older patients, in whom it improves nutrition, relieves emotional tension and mildly sedates.
8. Wine, used as a food with other foods at mealtimes, may play a vital role in developing a cultural or sociological protective pattern against excessive drinking.

Many physicians recommend judicious use of alcohol as an aid to making life more enjoyable for untold numbers of elderly people in the nation's nursing homes, hospitals, and private homes. Not only are fresh, dried and fermented grapes useful healthwise, but also the woody vine itself, whose spring sap has been drunk to clear up diarrhea, and applied to eye and skin infections. Travelers, troops on the march, and outdoorsmen have chewed on wild grape leaves to control diarrhea.

The grape plant contains minerals, vitamins (A, B_1, B_2, C), fruit acids and sugars, flavonoids, tannin, xanthophyll, gums, and laxative tartrates.

A stimulating Amazonian tea for fever, diarrhea, urinary inflammation, and headaches

Guarana (*Paullinia cupana*) seeds, named after the South American Guaraní Indians, who used to collect the seeds in the Amazon, promote urinary flow and reinforce the flushing effect of goldenrod when used in the same remedy. Guarana tea, brewed from crushed seeds and drunk regularly by millions of Amazonian inhabitants in town and jungle, has also been used by Amazonian Indians as a stimulant before combat and to prevent fever.

Guarana is drunk specifically as a remedy for diarrhea and dysentery, inflamed urinary passages (such as urethrifis), neuralgia, menstrual headache, and hangover headache.

Caffeine, tannin, and saponin are Guarana's main ingredients. Another South American tea, maté (*Ilex paraguensis*), which also contains caffeine and tannin, is an everyday beverage all over the continent, and makes a healthful and stimulating alternative to coffee. If you'd like to avoid all caffeine, however, try some of the other drinks mentioned in this book, such as caffeine-free chicory root and dandelion root "coffees," or the masai tea described below.

Other health-promoting tea-time beverages to replace black tea and coffee

Indian kidney tea (Orthsiphon stamineus)

When I first tried Indian kidney tea, I asked my tea-time hostess why it smelled faintly of urine. She not only didn't know why, but was somewhat insulted by my question. In the laboratory later, I learned that the plant contained urea (along with saponins, ethereal oil, a bitter glycoside, tannins, and potassium). And that made me happy, for urea is good for the teeth (that's why they put it in some dentrifices), so a cup of Indian kidney tea helped my teeth as well as my urinary system. As its name implies, Indian kidney tea (also called Java tea and long-stamened orthosiphon) promotes the flow of urine and clarifies it, including an increased excretion of uric acid. It has also been reported to extend the effect of insulin.

Some Europeans brew the tea as usual, steeping 10 minutes. A

German lawyer, however, told me he soaked 2 teaspoonsful of the leaves in a pint of cold water overnight, then took swallows of it throughout the day to allay the distress caused by his kidney stones, the tea helped most when he drank it just before a bout, when he felt it coming on. His winter rheumatism, too, the lawyer said, also seemed to let up and not bother him as much when he was drinking the tea.

The long stamens of the Indian kidney tea flowers look like cat whiskers, at least to the Malayan and Dutch growers in the East Indies, who called the plant *koemis koetjing*, which means cat whisker, and who supplied the leaves to the tea trade.

Masai or rooi tea (Aspalathus linearis)

Rooi is Afrikaans for *red*, which is the color of the brewed tea, and *Masai* is the name of a people native to East Africa. Both of these names refer to the same tea, one rich in minerals (aluminum, iron, calcium, magnesium, manganese, phosphorus, sulfur, potassium, sodium) and vitamin C. Research in South Africa showed, too, that Masaï tea contains 1% tannin, which is only a third of the 3% in ordinary tea.

An anti-diarrheal plant with twice the vitamin C of oranges, and a related fruit that eased a prolapsed anus

The guava (*Psidium guava*) probably gets its name from *gahyaba*, a Peruvian Indian word which came to us via the Spanish name for guava, *guayaba*. The *Psidium* part of guava's scientific name is from the Greek word *psidion* for *pomegranate*, because both the guava and its relative the pomegranate are filled with pulp-covered seeds from which you suck off the delicious pulp before either swallowing or spitting out the seeds. Guava fruit contains more than double the amount of vitamin C in oranges, and the tannin in various other parts of the guava plant makes it a useful remedy for diarrhea.

Pomegranates (*Punica granatum*), too, are an antidiarrheal remedy. The pomegranate's dried stem or root bark contains alkaloids and about 20% tannin; pomegranate's fruit rind contains about 30% tannin, all of which is puckeringly obvious to anyone who bites into the rind or the cabbage-looking partitions that enclose the glistening red fleshy seeds in the fruit.

A Japanese subway employee eased his prolapsed anus by applying strongly astringent wet compresses soaked in some alum and a strong tea made by boiling pomegranate rind, rootbark, and/or stems until about half of the water evaporated. The drawing or astringent effect usually helped relieve the distress by the time the sufferer settled down to sleep. At times, he inserted the lubricated tip of a cone-shaped paper cup and gently urged the extruding rectum back in through the muscular ring that forms the anus. Also, he was able to relieve his condition by using some of the hemorrhoidal remedies that reduce inflammation and act astringently.

Concerning guava in combination remedies, the World Health Organization reported from Ghana, Africa, that herpes zoster or shingles (which, incidentally, is caused by a virus apparently identical to that which causes chicken pox) is healed in about 10 days when the patient is treated twice a day with a paste of pounded guava leaves + kaolin (white clay from which fine Chinese porcelain is made) + Guinea pepper (*Piper guineense*).

How a businessman, a roofer, a physician and stressed diplomats benefited from a tree that stabilizes blood pressure, dissolves deposits in thickened arteries, and alleviates nervous heart ailments

Hawthorn (*Crataegus oxyacantha*) improves blood circulation, leading to more efficient oxygenation of the blood and tissues. Hawthorn unstresses and protectively tranquilizes the nervous system, strengthening the heart and stabilizing blood pressure within normal limits. This plant reportedly is capable of dissolving deposits in thickened or sclerotic arteries. All of these effects explain why hawthorn is one of the most important ingredients of herbal combination remedies for the heart. Such remedies protect the aging heart against myocardial infarction, coronary insufficiency, and disordered heart beat and rhythm. Hawthorn, too, is often used to alleviate nervous palpitations, anginal pain, and sleeplessness. Long-term use of hawthorn leads to measurable improvement in heart function. If however, you don't have any heart problem, then hawthorn protectively strengthens heart function and wards off potential problems.

Hawthorn contains flavonoids, tannins, coumarin, vitamins (B_1, C, niacin), pectin, pigments, the enzyme lipase, and other substances that contribute to its beneficial effects on the cardiovascular system.

A resident of the island of Jersey (in the English channel) sipped hawthorn tea he made by pouring 1 cupful of boiling water over 2 teaspoonsful of dried hawthorn flowers and steeping it 5 minutes. Several cupfuls a week allayed his nervous palpitations and the pains that radiated through his left arm whenever he felt overstressed with family and business problems.

A German-American roof estimator brewed hawthorn tea by soaking 2 teaspoonsful of mashed hawthorn berries in 1 cup of cold water overnight, then brought it to a boil in the morning before straining out the berries. A daily cup of this tea helped him to sleep nights and literally "took a load off" his heart by normalizing his blood pressure and quietening his pounding heart (caused by all the squabbling over prices in his estimates, and the litigation that followed unfortunate "roof deals" that didn't hold up under Florida heat and hurricanes).

How a plasterer relieved his hemorrhoidal discomfort with a tree whose nuts calm quivering eyelids and improve venous blood flow

Besides speeding up blood circulation, especially through the veins, horse chestnut (*Aesculus hippocastanum*) also specifically acts on the vein walls to shrink varicose veins, whether they be in the legs or in the rectum (where varicose veins are called hemorrhoids). There even seems to be an anesthetic effect in horse chestnuts that eases pains. The improved circulation, along with the effect of aesculin (a saponin also found in hawthorn, among other plants) relieves edema or water build-up in the tissues, and also relieves inflammation. Tests have shown horse chestnut's helpfulness in reducing post-stroke cerebral swelling. Horse chestnuts help clear up "wet" coughs, thanks in part to the expectorant effect of saponin. Horse chestnut liniment relieves gouty and rheumatic aches; in India, a poultice of the Himalayan horse chestnut is applied to the skin to alleviate the aches and pains of rheumatism. And, as an additional benefit, horse chestnut snuff calms down quivering eyelids!

In addition to the saponin aesculin mentioned above, the various organs of the horse chestnut tree (bark, flowers, seeds or nuts, leaves) also contain coumarin, flavonoids, tannin, resin, starch, guanine, vitamins (B_1, C and K), pigments, gums, phosphorus compounds, and other substances which, all together, account for the properties of this plant. Roasting appears to eliminate any toxins in the raw chestnuts.

A Chicago German-American plasterer relieved varicosed rectal veins (hemorrhoids) by taking a bath in which he poured a "tea" he brewed by boiling 2 to 3 pounds of diced horse chestnuts and a handful of bark he peeled from the tree's larger branches in enough water to cover them. Once he added the tree's leaves, too, and obtained so much "shrinkage" that his external hemorrhoids felt tight and ached so much that he got out of the bath, rinsed off and went right to bed, soon after which he fell asleep. When he awoke next morning, his hemorrhoids were reduced so much that when he moved his bowels he realized that swelling and inflammation were completely gone, that is, he couldn't feel his hemorrhoids any more. The last I heard from the plasterer, he hadn't had any more hemorrhoids, and that was almost seven months after his horse chestnut bath. Of course, some of the credit probably must go to other things, too, such as how carefully he began to avoid constipation, certain foods and prolonged standing, all of which no doubt helped him keep the overnight alleviation provided by the horse chestnut bath.

A white-flowered plant that relieved
a pharmacist's jaundice

Hoarhound or horehound (*Marrubium vulgare*) is named from the Anglo-Saxon words *har* (gray) plus *hune* (hound) because the grayish felt covering of the plant's branches resembled the coat of a particular breed of dog. Hoarhound foliage helps bring up phlegm, aids digestion, improves liver and gallbladder function, and helps control irregularities of heart rhythm. Hot hoarhound tea has sweated out many a cold, soothed many an inflamed and irritated throat, and relieved many a cough.

Marrubin, one of the bitter principles in hoarhound, is mainly responsible for stimulating secretion along the respiratory tract so the phlegm can be cleared out, thus easing breathing and alleviating bronchitic distress. Hoarhound's effects also involve other bitters as well as tannin, ethereal oil, resins, vitamin C, and perhaps an alkaloid whose presence may be more widespread in some hoarhound plants than in others. The reason is that plants, like people, often reflect their environment, and contain variable quantities of a substance, or even totally different substances, depending upon the nutrients or the lack of them in the soil where the plants were grown.

For clearing up his jaundice, a pharmacist in Syracuse, New York, brewed a gallbladder and liver tea (20 grams of hoarhound foliage to 6 or 7 ounces of water) which he drank cold during the day in 3 portions of about 2 ounces each time.

A sedative, antimicrobial plant an old doctor
used to relieve alcoholic "jeebies"

Hops (*Humulus lupulus* or *Cannabis lupulus*) gets its English name from Anglo-Saxon *hoppen* (meaning *to climb*) because of its habit of sending out runners or vines. The mildly sedative effect of hops is obvious to anyone who enjoys beer. Hops can take the edge off of sexual interest, that is, it's an anaphrodisiac. Poorly healing wounds often improve after treatment with hops extract, which is antimicrobial. A large part of hops is a bitter resin; its other ingredients include ethereal oil (which in turn contains about 200 aromatic compounds!), bitters, tannin, flavonoids, asparagine (a growth-promoting amino acid), hopein (an alkaloid-like substance with narcotic effect), and substances with estrogenic effects. Hops, by the way, is related to *Cannabis indica,* the source of marihuana.

If you like beer, then hops certainly has its calling as part of this medicinally valuable beverage, especially where beer is brewed naturally and contains *only* good water, malt and hops. Bavaria is one such place, and there are others, but not many.

If you don't care for beer, then hops tea or baths made from the female catkins or from an extract of hops, can also be useful to chase insomnia, tension, nervousness, menopausal distress, and migraine.

Hops as a remedy is not recommended in cases of mental depression. It should also be mentioned that some people reportedly had allergic reactions to *fresh* hops plants, so sensitive individuals might prefer dried hops or extracts or the plant, rather than the fresh catkins.

A very old Philadelphia doctor prescribed hops tea for his patients with delirium tremens, to quieten the craving for drink and to settle the stomach. He had some of his patients inhale the vapor of boiling hops for throat and chest conditions. Also, he applied hops poultices to relieve painful inflammations.

A silicon-rich diuretic plant for the lungs, gout, bleeding, wounds..., and for scouring utensils and polishing wood

The horsetail (*Equisetum arvense* and other species) is called that because it looks somewhat like a horse's tail, at least to the settlers who named it that, and who also called it *scouring rush* (because the silicon particles in it made it useful in cleaning and shining up metalware before the days of Brillo and Bon Ami), and who also called it *shavegrass* (because they used it, too, for sanding wood). The silicon-containing compounds, along with aluminum, calcium, flavonoids, saponin, bitter principles, resin, alkaloids, and other substances account for horsetail's favorable effects on certain forms of pulmonary tuberculosis, hemorrhage-arresting effects (that help control nasal, lung, stomach, bladder, and uterine bleeding), stimulation of urinary flow, encouragement of tissue elasticity and resilience, and stepping up of resistance. (See also the narrow-leaved purple coneflower for another resistance-building plant.)

Horsetail baths are used to relieve neuralgia, rheumatism, gout, neurodermatitis, eczema, and post-thrombotic swellings. To prepare a bath, pour a gallon of boiling water over 150 grams of horsetail foliage, steep 10 minutes, then add it to the bathwater.

Horsetail wet dressings made with the above gallon (or portion thereof) of bath solution, can be applied over eczema and other skin conditions that might benefit from horsetail.

Horsetail gargle, made by pouring a cup of boiling water over a teaspoonful of dried foliage, can ease tonsilitis, the soreness of gum recession, and the distress of carious teeth (but not as well in some cases as a few drops of clove oil).

How a rural nurse alleviated chronic diarrhea with a nutritional anti-tubercular lichen

Iceland moss (*Cetraria islandica*) is really a lichen—a permanent combination of a fungus with an alga—that contains carbohydrates, vitamin A, iodine (but only in Iceland moss grown near the ocean), mucilage and bitters (but boiling takes away the bitterness), and lichenic acids, at least one of which arrests or retards tuberculosis. These ingredients explain many of Iceland moss's uses, which include sparking the appetite of convalescents or others suffering from malnutrition, soothing irritated respiratory passages and gastrointestinal tissues, alleviating vomiting, and encouraging the flow of milk in nursing mothers (but it's not used for this purpose if the mother's nipples or breasts are inflamed).

Nutritious Iceland moss was also used to fatten up hogs in the Alpine farming community I found after a five-hour hike from the closest Bavarian village. Horse enthusiasts of a certain age will remember the thoroughbred Sea Biscuit, who was named after the synonym for the hardtack or ship biscuit of pre-refrigeration sailing days. That biscuit was baked with Iceland moss in it to retard spoilage and ward off weevil attack during long ocean voyages. Diabetic bread, too, has been made from Iceland moss because a large proportion of its carbohydrate (galactose and mannose) content is easily resorbed.

A rural Norweigian nurse used 15 to 30 grams of a decoction (1 part of Iceland moss boiled in 10 to 15 parts of water) for chronic diarrhea in debilitated patients. She either gave it as a sweetened tea, or by the spoonful.

How a lumberman, a doctor, a ship chandler and a pharmacist used gin berries to ease rheumatism, neuralgia, bronchitis, and indigestion

Juniper (*Juniperus communis*), the berry plant that became famous as the source of gin, is an evergreen shrub that grows to about six feet, or a tree that can grow to well over thirty feet. Although the use of juniper berries to flavor gin and other alcoholic beverages made people more aware of the juniper plant's existence, the plant was already known well enough for its curative properties long before the Dutch made gin from them.

Some scholars say that juniper's scientific name, *Juniperus*, may come from the Latin *junior* (the younger) plus *pario* (to appear or be born), referring to the appearance of the immature, green fruit even while the older, blue-black ones are still hanging on the branches. (Juniper berries stay green the first year, then ripen and darken during the second autumn). Other scholars say that *Juniperus* comes from the Celtic word *jeneprus*, referring to the plant's prickly leaves or perhaps to the tart, pungent taste of the berries.

Besides the pleasant aroma and taste that juniper's ethereal oil gives to alcoholic drinks, this oil, along with flavonoids, tannin, resin and other substances, accounts for the effect of juniper in natural remedies to disinfect the urine and promote its flow (especially of its sodium and chloride components) in persons suffering from bladder infections (but free of inflammatory kidney problems), chronic neuralgia, and the distress caused by gout, rheumatism, and arthritis. A North Carolina lumberman rubbed a few crushed juniper berries into his skin to alleviate neuralgic and rheumatic aches, and also dropped a handful of crushed berries into his bathwater for the same relief. (An old Alpine doctor once said that juniper berry baths and compresses are the ultimate hope for rheumatic stiffness in the elderly.) Juniper also enhances stomach tone and function, and allays digestive distress by expelling or preventing gas and calming cramping ... and that is why some European cooks put juniper berries into their cabbage, sauerkraut, and other foods that tend to create some gas in certain people.

Juniper has also been useful in relieving bronchitis and other chest distress; a Norwegian ship chandler eased his respiratory infection by inhaling juniper berry vapors (handful of crushed berries in a kettle of boiling water), and drinking hot linden blossom tea. Watch out for the invisible live steam between the spout and the cloud of visible steam or vapor over a kettle or pan of boiling water. It might even be safer to inhale the vapors after you've taken the kettle off the heat; the ethereal oil vapors will be strong enough to smell even if the water is not actually boiling.

The wood shavings from juniper heartwood (from another species of juniper) are distilled to manufacture juniper tar, which is used in ointments for clearing up eczema, scabies and various other skin conditions.

For his digestive problems, a Hamburg pharmacist chewed up 5 to 10 dried juniper berries a day, a few before each meal. For his urinary and rheumatic problems, he drank 2 cups a day of juniper tea made by pouring 2 cups of boiling water over 100 grams of crushed juniper berries, and steeping it about 20 minutes. Or, he poured 1 cupful of boiling water over 1 tablespoonful of crushed dried berries, steeped it in a covered cup for about 10 minutes, then sipped half a cup, or even up to 1 cup a day, which he didn't sweeten when he was drinking it for his digestion.

Note: Don't confuse wholesome, aromatic *Juniper communis* with toxic and abortifacient *Juniperus sabina*, whose unpleasant smell led to one of its German names, *Stinkwacholder* or stinking juniper. Too much of even a good kind, by the way, could cause uterine contractions, so expectant mothers should be careful when using it, or when using any medicines for that matter. Juniper berries are not recommended for persons suffering from acute kidney inflammation.

A Cree Indian tea that eased a bush pilot's burns, wounds, and arthritis

The Cree Indians chewed Labrador tea (*Ledum palustre*, also called marsh tea or wild rosemary) leaves into a wad and packed it over their burns, quite an understandable use for a plant that contains tannin—a substance found in some burn ointments (but not recommended any more for serious burns). Labrador tea also contains ethereal oil, bitter principles, arbutin glycoside, a flavonoid, resin, and other substances that contribute to the plant's use for promoting urinary flow, clearing out phlegm from the throat and chest, and alleviating rheumatism and gout. Another name for Labrador tea, *brewer's tea*, refers to the use of this plant for stepping up the euphoric or "happy" effect of beer. Still another name, *moth herb*, refers to its use in getting rid of moths and other tiny vermin.

For getting phlegm up and easing his minor arthritic aches, a Canadian bush pilot soaked 2 tablespoonsful of crushed dried Labrador tea foliage and leaves in a cup of cold water overnight. Then he drank half a cupful (but not more) during the next day. He saved the other half a cupful to swab over any little burns or skin wounds he picked up during the next day or two, and he even applied the soggy wad of soaked-out leaves over his burns to relieve the pain and hasten their healing, just like the Cree Indians used the leaves.

Fragrant flowers that sedate, alleviate migraine, and chase vermin

Lavender's name (*Lavandula officinalis*) comes from the Latin *lavere* (meaning *to wash*) because of its frequent use in baths (lavender flower tea added to bathwater) to mildly sedate the central nervous system just to the point of letting you breathe easily and feel relaxed, just as Rose B. did every week by dumping 1 to 2 cupsful of strong lavender flower tea into her warm bath. This sedative bath (which was all the perfuming Rose ever used—and she was as sweet-scented as her name) calmed down her heart palpitations and settled her nerves.

Tea prepared in the usual manner (boiling water poured over plant parts) from lavender flowers relieves gastrointestinal distress by stimulating digestion (especially gallbladder function), prevents and expels gas, and dispels the uneasy feeling of fulness after eating.

Lavender flowers in teas and baths also alleviate migraine headaches and chase away tiny vermin. King Charles VI of France enjoyed satin cushions filled with fragrant lavender, but the historian who chronicled that bit of information carefully avoided any reference to either the king's headaches or to any vermin in the royal chambers. Besides ethereal oil, the tannin and various other substances in lavender account for all the above effects.

How a botany teacher eased hoarseness and coughs with a steroid-like anti-inflammatory, anti-cramping candy-flavoring root

Licorice's English name as well as its Latin scientific name (*Glycyrrhiza glabra*), are still quite similar to its medieval name *gliquiricia*, which comes from Greek *glykos* (sweet) plus *riza* (root), all of which alludes to the sweet taste of licorice root . . . which is 40 to 150 times sweeter than sugar. The German word for licorice, in fact, is *Süssholz*, literally *sweet wood*, a term still used by some English-speaking pharmacists.

Licorice soothes inflamed gastrointestinal.tissues, relieves cramping, gets phlegm up and out, and alleviates hoarseness. Licorice's anti-inflammatory effect on the lining of the respiratory passages has been attributed to a steroid-like action similar to that of a hormone from the adrenal gland. The calcium in licorice no doubt contributes to the anti-inflammatory effect.

Licorice is an ingredient of "Brown's mixture," which you may remember being given as a child to quickly ease "wet" coughs by helping you to get the phlegm up and out—an effect due to the saponin-like glycyrrhicin (a calcium and potassium compound) in licorice. This effect is supported by other substances in licorice such as bitters, resin, the amino acid asparagine, and flavonoids.

Note: In some people under some conditions, excessive eating of licorice candy (say about 20 grams or more) can raise the blood pressure, weaken muscles, and lead to sodium retention and edema. Persons with high blood pressure and related cardiovascular conditions, fluid and ionic imbalances, bleeding ulcers, or kidney disease should check with their doctors before consuming too much licorice.

A Honolulu botany professor always found immediate relief for his and his wife's hoarseness and coughs (which they picked up whenever they attended professional congresses in cold and wet cities on the U.S. mainland) by drinking a tea made by boiling 1 teaspoonful of diced dried licorice root in 1 cup of water for about 10 minutes.

An alert Hong Kong policeman often prevented disaster in the crowded dock areas by beating out small blazes with his feet and hands. For easing his minor burns and hastening their healing, he applied compresses soaked in water in which he had boiled ginseng (*Panax ginseng*) and a Chinese species of licorice (*Glycyrrhiza uralensis*).

A flower that sweats out colds, eases digestive distress, and allays migraine and arteriosclerotic hypertension

In Germany, the village linden tree (*Tilia* species) stands in special esteem. The linden or basswood tree, also called lime (but not the citrus kind), contains mucilage, vitamin E, ethereal oil, flavonoids, tannin, perhaps saponins, and other substances that contribute to its use in soothing the lining of the respiratory passages, sweating out colds, alleviating cramps, promoting bile secretion, soothing of wounds, and caring for the skin. Linden is often combined with sage to quiet convulsive coughing; with peppermint it alleviates wet coughs, colds, gas, cramps, enteritis, neuralgia, rheumatism, and headache; with elder and mullein it sweats out colds. Linden flower tea is drunk in Europe by people who suffer from arteriosclerotic high blood pressure and nervousness. Linden bark contains a cramp-relieving substance, and charcoal from the wood has eased chronic skin conditions, wounds, acid stomach, and diarrhea.

Hot linden blossom tea (brewed by pouring 1 cupful of boiling water over 2 teaspoonsful of flowers and steeping 10 minutes before straining out the flowers) is a popular European remedy—1 to 2 cups a day—for colds, gastrointestinal and urinary tract cramps, as well as nervousness.

A spice that eases gas and phlegm

Lovage's name (*Levisticum officinale*) comes from old English *lufestice* and Anglo-French *luvesche*, which shows that it was around a long time before the Norman invasion of England in 1066, and stayed on to become part of the new England under William the Conqueror. Besides helping digestion when used as a spice in cooking, lovage (root, foliage, seed-like fruit) also promotes the flow of urine, expels gas, and frees the respiratory passages by helping to clear out any accumulated phlegm.

Ten days after Paul S. began adding pinches of lovage to his daily soup, salads and meats, his bronchial, asthmatic-like phlegm problem started to clear up, giving him easier breathing. Paul's wife stopped her gas problem by alternating lovage with other anti-gas spices in her food.

Although spices and other plants also have many *immediate* effects towards better health, one should not overlook the fact that such plants are used *dietarily* worldwide for *preventing* little (and some not so little) discomforts (gas, etc.), so are not always thought of as outright remedies, but as *protectors*.

Lovage's parts contain ethereal oil, resin, coumarin derivatives, bitters, and other substances that account for lovage's effects.

A dye root that prevented and may also have actually dissolved an artist's calcium phosphate urinary stones

An Italian artist who still grinds and mixes his own pigments laughed when I asked if his colleagues made fun of his not buying ready-made tube paints. "Certainly not," he assured me, "because my artist friends who suffer from urinary stones come to me for some of my madder root powder!"

Madder root is a natural source of important alizarin dyes such as turkey red. The natural dyes in an older madder (*Rubia tinctorum*) root—a natural source of industrially important alizarin dyes such as turkey red—along with its other ingredients (tannins, anthraquinones, enzymes, pectin, etc.), exert anti-inflammatory and cramp-relieving effects on the kidney and the rest of the urinary system, especially relaxation of the ureter muscle, thus letting stones work themselves down easier and with less pain. (Madder root colors your urine red, so don't panic when you see it.) Madder prevents the formation of calcium phosphate stones and may also be able to dissolve them because the dyes form a soluble compound with the calcium, thus allowing them to be excreted with the urine. This root, too, has been useful in clearing up diarrhea and intestinal infections, as well as healing throat and skin ulcers and other wounds.

The artist's ailing fellow painters soaked 1 teaspoonful of crushed and ground madder root in 1 cup of cold water overnight, brought it to a boil the next morning, and then drank a cup of it warm to alleviate their phosphate and urate stone problems. They drank a cup or two of the madder root tea as a preventive measure, but also to relieve an attack once it started.

An Asiatic anti-asthma and anti-tubercular nut tree that eases breathing

Leaves of the Malabar nut or adhatoda tree (*Adhatoda vasica*) promote the clearing of secretions and phlegm from the respiratory passages. To breathe more easily, asthmatics and sufferers of chronic bronchitis have smoked adhatoda leaves as cigarettes, taken them as powders, or drunk them as tinctures. Among other substances, adhatoda contains alkaloids and an ethereal oil with anti-tubercular activity.

Mallow and marshmallow—two softeners that soothe irritated and inflamed tissues

Because of the possible confusion between two similarly named and similarly acting plants—mallow and marshmallow—I've briefly compared their characteristics, properties, and uses in the following table:

	Mallow (*Malva sylvestris, Malva neglecta*)	Marshmallow (*Althaea officinalis*)
Appearance	5 light carmine heart-shaped petals. Leaves palmate with 5 to 7 lobes	5 pinkish white heart-shaped petals. Leaves may be heart-shaped with 3 to 7 lobes.
Parts used	Flowers, leaves, foliage	Root, leaves, flowers
Content	Anthrocyanglycoside in the flowers, tannin in the leaves, and a great deal of mucilage in all parts	Mucilage in all parts, especially in the winter roots. Pectin, starch, asparagine, a little ethereal oil, tannin, phosphates
Properties	Reduces irritation and inflammation. Leaves are mildly astringent.	Protects mucous membranes, reduces irritation, relieves coughing, promotes healthy blood coagulation.
Uses	A tea for gargling (5 times a day), for an eyewash or for wet dressings can be made by pouring a cupful of boiling water over 1 to 2 teaspoonsful of foliage and flowers, bringing it to a boil, then steeping it 5 minutes before straining out the plant parts. Use for sores, abscesses, gum boils, hemorrhoids, sore throats, inflamed eyelids.	Soak a tablespoonful of chopped root about 5 hours. Then use 1 or 2 teaspoonsful with 1 teaspoonful of honey hourly for easing bronchitis coughs, hoarseness, sore throat. Several spoonsful (but without honey) every 2 hours soothes gastro-enteritis. Grated root mixed with honey makes a soothing poultice to apply about every 3 hours on skin conditions.

A European geriatric strengthening tea is made by soaking 1 tablespoonful of marshmallow (assorted parts cut up finely) 15 minutes in half a pint of cool water. If mucus is also present in the respiratory passages, then plantain foliage, coltsfoot leaves, and Iceland moss are added to loosen up the mucus more effectively.

Both mallow and marshmallow are combined to make the following tea; rinse or dressing for soothing and hastening the healing of irritated, inflamed tissues:

  1 part marshmallow leaves
  1 part mallow leaves
  1 part melilot foliage
  1 part camomile flowers
  1 part linseed (crushed)

How a chemist mixed an ointment
from an orange-yellow flower
for skin care and healing wounds

The name marigold (*Calendula officinalis*) is from *Mary* and from the flower's golden yellow color—once used as a dye. The name calendula may come from the Latin word for the first day of the month (*kalendae*) because the plant flowers almost monthly. Marigold's xanthophyll and other carotinoids (which create the flower's rich golden color), saponins, mucilage, resin and gum, bitters, enzymes, ethereal oil, salicylic acid, and other substances account for many of its effects, often quite similar to those of arnica. Marigold can be used for sebaceous cysts and inflamed sores, purulent gaping wounds, and other wounds in which arnica would be too strong (and would irritate further). Fresh marigold sap has been rubbed on warts regularly to eliminate them (but I don't have any report yet on how long that takes).

Indolent ulcers of the legs and other poorly healing wounds are often helped by marigold ointment, which prevents inflammation and hastens the formation of scabs. To make an ointment, an Irish chemist recommended the following: heat 1 ounce of clean lard, lanolin, or petroleum jelly with 1 ounce of dried marigold leaves and/or flowers. When the mix boils, let it simmer a few moments, then strain it through clean cheesecloth or gauze, and there you have a pomade or ointment to apply to wounds and sores.

Another way to make a marigold salve is to boil the leaves and flowers about 10 minutes in water, strain out and discard the plant debris, pour this tea you just made into olive or other good food-quality oil, and heat until the water evaporates, thus transferring the plant's natural chemical substances from the water to the oil. A professional pharmacist who compounds an ointment or salve like this may also add some melted beeswax to stiffen the mix so that it sticks to where you apply it, and doesn't drip away too rapidly.

A reminder about getting at skin ailments from inside the body: The above externally applied salve is good for various skin conditions. Drinking the marigold, however, can also help clear up skin problems such as abscesses and boils. As explained elsewhere in this book, you can often get at skin ailments *from the inside* by drinking spring tonics and blood-cleansing teas.

Marigold tea can be made by pouring 1 cup of boiling water over several tablespoonsful of dried marigold flowers, steeping about 10 minutes, and then straining out the plant parts. About 1 table-spoonful of this tea hourly has helped not only gallbladder sufferers to control cramping, but also has eased gastrointestinal distress, including diarrhea and nausea.

How an accountant healed his wounds with a clover that also loosens blood clots

Melilot or yellow sweet clover (*Melilotus officinalis*) gets it name from a Greek word for honey lotus, which was a name for clover among the ancient Greeks. Various species of melilot are the source of a drug used medically to prevent or to dissolve the clotting of blood in the heart, arteries, veins and capillaries. Melilot's aromatic powers make it a useful addition to other, stronger-tasting plants used in combination remedies. This clover has also been used to relieve cramping and to add to dressings put on running, pus-filled wounds and sores. Here is how a rural accountant made a dressing to heal his festered wound caused by a fish hook: he filled a small, cleanly laundered white sock with an ounce or so of dried melilot foliage, that is, the above-ground parts of the plant, and boiled the filled sock in a pot of water for a moment. He let it cool down only enough until he was able to tolerate it on his wound and surrounding skin, then he covered the wound with the hot, sopping wet sock for 30 to 60 minutes, depending upon how long it took to get cold. His wounds always healed cleanly with minimal pain (if any), usually within a week or so.

The doctor down the road said antibiotics wouldn't have done any better. He also suggested that the accountant ease his next charley horse or sprain with a pinch of melilot foliage mixed with a handful of hay bloom (that is, all those miscellaneous bits and pieces of field flowers and hay particles left over from a load of hay) in a clean sock, all of which is moistened with steam, then squeezed out and placed over the injury for about 45 minutes.

Clover tea, too, helped as a wet dressing. The accountant poured 1 cupful of boiling water over 1 teaspoonful of dried melilot foliage, then steeped it for 5 to 10 minutes before straining out the plant parts and soaking his compresses in the tea.

Melilot contains, among other substances, coumarin, purine derivatives, mucilage, amino acids, tannins, flavonoids, and ethereal oil.

A digestive, anti-bleeding plant known to the ancient world

Milfoil or yarrow (*Achillea millefolium*) gets its English name from its Latin scientific name *millefolium* (thousand leaf) referring to the plant's finely divided feather-like leaves. The *Achillea* part of the scientific name comes from Achilles, who was the first to use this plant medicinally, as Pliny tells us in his ancient writings. Icelanders of the middle ages brewed their beer with milfoil, which they called "field hops."

Milfoil's antiseptic ethereal oil, astringent tannins, digestion-stimulating bitters, inulin, ascorbic acid, antibiotic substances, flavonoids, aspirin-like salicylic acid, resin, amino acids, prussic acid, alkaloids, and other substances account for the plant's usefulness.

Besides milfoil's general help to digestion and appetite, it promotes healthy gallbladder function. Its antiseptic properties prevent urinary and respiratory infections. Long term use of milfoil lessens the bleeding problems of hemorrhoids, bladder, uterus, intestines, and lungs. This hemorrhage-arresting effect is responsible for yet another name for the plant: *nosebleed. Soldier's woundwort*, too, is still another name for milfoil that refers to its use in the past.

Prepare a tea in the standard way (that is, pour 1 cup of boiling water over 1 tablespoonful of milfoil flowers and steep 10 minutes), but don't overuse it, for it may make the skin of some persons temporarily overly sensitive to sunlight, just as Saint John's wort may do, too.

The heart-protecting, anti-hypertensive and anti-tumor properties of the magical plant of the ancient Druids

Amid the sacrifice of victims and the fasting of cult members in ancient Britain, a Druid priest in white robes cut European mistletoe (*Viscum album*) with a golden sickle, then distributed it as a heal-all, a charm against disaster, and a symbol of fertility. A recent U.S. committee of experts who visited the People's Republic of China reported that mistletoe was being used there to slow the pulse and calm down heart action as well as to reduce inflammation in various parts of the body. The Chinese also used mistletoe against cancer, a use supported by western scientific studies that demonstrate well enough the favorable effect of mistletoe extract on tumors and cancers in animals. Europeans use mistletoe for protection against arteriosclerotic problems (dizziness, lethargy, restlessness, and fluctuations in circulation), and the maintenance of normal blood pressure within accustomed limits. Mistletoe leaves reportedly stimulate some metabolic and glandular activity.

European mistletoe cqntains amino acids, cardioactive viscotoxin, various substances that reduce blood pressure (butyric acid, etc.), a tumor-inhibiting and resistance-increasing substance, inositol, flavonoids, mucilage and other substances. The berries of both kinds of mistletoe—the European and the American—are toxic, so don't use them. The leafy stems (twigs and leaves) are soaked in cold water (1 teaspoonful chopped stems in 1 cup of water) a whole day and night, the resulting tea being drunk in thirds over the following day. Or the leaves can be soaked overnight. A representative package of mistletoe leaves sold on the European market advises one to pour 1 cupful of boiling water over 1 teaspoonful of the dried leaves and steep 5 to 10 minutes; the package says the tea is for high blood pressure, fluctuations in circulation, dizziness, and hardening of the arteries. In any case, however, like some of the other cardioactive plants mentioned in this book, it's best to use such plants only in professionally prepared remedies, preferably with your physician's help.

Note: Avoid American mistletoe entirely. The leaves, stems and berries are toxic, as are the berries of the European mistletoe.

Another cardioactive plant, mossy stonecrop (*Sedum acre*), by the way, widens blood vessels and lowers blood pressure. Mossy stonecrop contains alkaloids, tannins, mucilage, gum, the flavonoid rutin, nicotine, fruit acids, and other substances that contribute to its effects on our health.

Mistletoe helps in the fight against tumors' spread

The anticancer use of mistletoe was explained to me by a physician of the Arlesheim Society for Cancer Research. One sunny Indian summer day in October I lunched with this physician at the hospital she directs. Her hospital, called a *clinic* here in the tidy Swiss village of Arlesheim (whose cathedral just celebrated its 300th anniversary, and in whose hills you can find traces of prehistoric cultures), specializes in therapy for tumor (cancer) sufferers. This highly individualized anticancer therapy provides a whole-person treatment built upon (1) modern medical methods used in any modern hospital, (2) mistletoe extract, (3) the whole-person anthroposophic approach to health and disease, and (4) lactovegetarian diet.

This tumor hospital is not a wonder-cure clinic, but is apparently successful in its use of natural products and forces (diet, mistletoe, and anthroposophic whole-person approach) to help post-surgical as well as inoperable patients.

About mistletoe in the total treatment of tumor or cancer victims, the hospital directress informed me that they followed up a group of patients who received Iscador (a mistletoe preparation) therapy soon after surgery and/or irradiation for tumors (cancers), and saw that after five years the death rate was much less than it was for patients who did not receive such therapy following surgery or irradiation. Mistletoe therapy was given after the tumor was surgically removed or destroyed by irradiation. The patient did not have a tumor any longer. The effect of the mistletoe treatment was that no new tumors occurred . . . a fact explained by the concept that tumors and cancers are not merely *local* diseases, but generalized ones. The directress also said:

"Patients with inoperable tumors often come to us. Within certain limits, they can be helped. Their general condition improves and only rarely are pain-relievers used. The spread of the disease can usually be slowed down, often held in check for years. Tumors may, in some cases, become smaller, occasionally disappearing completely. At times, it is especially impressive to see how new tumors develop if the therapy is interrupted . . . but regress once therapy starts again."

Such medication with mistletoe, of course, is not a casual home remedy, but requires experienced medical application.

How yellow flowers and flannel-like leaves mollify cough-irritated tissues

Mullein or flannel flower plant (*Verbascum thapsiforme*) gets its name from middle English *moleine*, which may come from the Latin word *moll(is)* for soft, an allusion to the ample content of "mollifying" mucilage in the plant, which soothes the tickling urge to cough. Besides mucilage, mullein flowers and leaves contain saponins, xanthophyll and other carotinoid pigments, flavonoids, ethereal oil, bitters, and other substances that account for the plant's other effects such as helping you to cough up and clear out phlegm. Another name for mullein, *cow's lungwort*, reveals that it was once used for treating cows for pulmonary diseases.

Powdered dried mullein leaves are sometimes sprinkled on poorly healing sores and wounds, just as European farmers and Andean

Indians do with powdered plantain leaves.

A recipe for a mildly laxative mullein tea that also stimulates the appetite of convalescents who feel too ill to eat, is made by adding 3 teaspoonsful of mullein flowers to 1 cupful of hot water and boiling for several minutes. Or the standard tea can be made by pouring 1 cupful of boiling water over a teaspoonful of mullein flowers and/or leaves and steeping about 5 minutes before straining out the plant parts, and drinking the tea warm, perhaps sweetened with a little honey if the tea is for a respiratory condition.

How mustard-oil plants eased chest pain, stopped hair loss, and relieved swollen testicles

The word *mustard* comes from Latin *mustum*, a mixture the Romans made by pounding mustard seeds with vinegar. Bengalese men rubbed mustard oil into their skin to soften, clean, and cool it before bathing, as well as to encourage their hair to grow. (Bengalese women, on the other hand, used coconut oil instead of mustard oil for cleaning their skin.) Too much mustard, of course, reddens and irritates the skin, yet is exactly what some sufferers do to relieve their rheumatism and neuralgia. They capitalize upon the principle of counter-irritation—the mustard stimulates the skin and improves local circulation of blood under it. This mild irritation not only lessens the underlying pain directly, but also serves to take the sufferer's attention away from the deeper pains, which, of course, is indirect, but does help—just like the rheumatic and arthritic victims who flog themselves with stinging nettle foliage for relief from their aches!

The local action of mustard on the skin, including its antibacterial properties, make it quite useful as a home remedy. Mustard plasters on the skin not only alleviate the distress of rheumatism and neuralgia, but also of neuritis, laryngitis, bronchitis, pneumonia, heart pains, headaches, chronic digestive upsets and nausea.

To make a mustard plaster, some people mix up as little as 4 to 6 tablespoonsful of ground black mustard (*Sinapsis nigra* or *Brassica nigra*), or as much as 100 grams of it, in enough lukewarm to hot water to make a paste, which they spread thinly over a clean linen cloth and lay over the skin until it feels like it's beginning to burn, which could be 5 to 10 minutes for some people. Some nurses rub olive or other good oil lightly over the skin before applying the mustard, and some rub it on after applying the mustard. Instead of oil, some people dust rice or rye flour on the skin before applying the mustard. In any case, the purpose of the oil or the flour is to protect delicate skin from too much irritation by the mustard. Cool water, too, can be sponged on the skin after the mustard plaster is removed.

Mustard plaster can provide immediate relief from the underlying pain of neuralgia and rheumatism; relief of respiratory conditions may take several plasters. One or so a day should be enough, for too many might burn the skin.

Taken internally, prepared condiment mustard aids digestion and improves appetite. One tablespoonful of powdered mustard in a glass of water has been taken to induce victims of certain kinds of poisoning to throw up the poison. On the other hand, too much can be dangerous, so don't ingest overly large amounts of mustard seed, mustard meal (that is, crushed seeds) or mustard oil.

White mustard (*Sinapsis alba* or *Brassica alba*) is used perhaps more in the kitchen for cooking than for plasters, although some people have mixed both mustards, the black and the white kinds, together for the above uses.

Other mustard oil plants such as horseradish and watercress also aid digestion. Watercress, by the way, is rich in vitamins (A, C and some D), and contains manganese as well as iodine. One investigator reported that he counteracted the effect of a lethal dose of nicotine in animals by treating them with the juice he squeezed from fresh watercress (*Nasturtium officinale*).

A Johannesburg merchant told me he used an old Boer settler's remedy to stop coughs: he poured honey over fresh, cut-up watercress and then left the mixture in his oven for about 8 hours. A few teaspoonsful of this honey-watercress mix stopped his coughing in 15-45 minutes, although I don't know what kind of cough it was (there are wet and dry ones, and various causes for coughing).

Another species of the *Brassica* genus, the turnip (*Brassica campestris*), is mashed up with fresh pink radishes (*Raphanus sativus*) in the Orient to make a poultice for sore testicles. For easing his painfully swollen and inflamed, heavy-feeling testicles, a Japanese bus driver applied this poultice, and enjoyed relief, he said, within an hour.

(Agricultural scientists learned that some plants, including turnips, which are sprayed with the ordinarily non-poisonous 2, 4-D contact herbicide may accumulate poisonous amounts of potassium nitrate. But that's a danger mainly for cattle who munch all day on plants.)

Here's another Oriental turnip remedy: A Chinese remedy for hair loss, particularly from other than just the natural balding process, is to pound fresh turnip seeds and mix them with vinegar. Strain out the mashed seeds and rub the liquid into the scalp 3 times a day. "It works from time to time in my family," was all the Chinese seaman who reported this told me about results.

A breakfast cereal that also lifts depression, dispels melancholy and helps skin ailments

Many people don't suspect that ordinary everyday oat (*Avena sativa*) grain and straw possess an anti-depression power which helps ease some menopausal problems and melancholy.

Dehusked oat seeds (or groats) when ground into meal and applied as a moist warm cataplasm to skin infections such as boils, encourage the escape of pus. Dry oatmeal has been sprinkled over running sores to absorb the wetness and promote healing.

How a waiter eased his aching corns with slices of an ordinary anti-blood-clotting, antimicrobial kitchen vegetable

Onion (*Allium cepa*), and its close relative garlic (*Allium sativum*), too, for that matter, are noble members of the lily family! This may surprise some people, but not the good cooks who lovingly speak of the *fragrance* and *perfume* of these two culinary gems. Scientific studies have already shown that people who enjoy onions and garlic regularly are usually better off for it. Garlic is discussed elsewhere in this book. As for onions, it was found that they increase the blood's ability to dissolve away dangerous blood clots—something long felt by folk instinct out in rural villages. Part of onion's beneficial effect on heart function may be due to its calcium and flavonoids.

Onions act antibacterially, promote the healing of wounds, and protect us from infections, especially respiratory ones. Onions promote the flow of urine and lower the amount of sugar in the blood. Part of this effect on sugar is due to glucokinine, an insulin-like hormone. Onions stimulate good digestion and build blood, that is, they supply minerals and vitamins needed for healthy blood, and they probably also directly bolster the blood-forming cells in the bone marrow. Onion, too, is used in hair-growth products.

Besides the glucokinine, cardioactive substances, flavonoids, vitamins (especially vitamin C), and minerals (especially calcium and sulfur), onions also contain enzymes, insulin, hormones which affect our gonads, and other substances. Even the most daring of cooks, however, might shy away from onions if they knew or had to remember that this vegetable contains compounds with names like 3-amino-3-carboxypropyldimethylsulfonium hydroxide!

A waiter from Hof, Germany, applied vinegar-soaked onion slices over his corns and left them on all night (by pulling a freshly laundered white sock over them to hold the slices in place). Several nights of this treatment either eased his aching toes or else softened the corns enough for him to peel some of them away.

An ornamental flower that alleviated a fertilizer salesman's eczema

Pansy or heart's ease (*Viola tricolor*) gets its name from the French *pensée*, which means *thought, reminiscence* or *sentiment,* alluding to this colorful flower's sentimental uses. Pansy is mainly known to apothecaries as a saponin plant for getting phlegm up and out, but its other constituents—the flavonoid rutin, some ethereal oil, mucilage, bitters, salicylic acid compounds, alkaloids, tannin, odoratin (a substance that lowers blood pressure), and pigment—

contribute to its other uses, which include promotion of urinary flow, sweating out of impurities, and alleviation of skin conditions, especially by purification of the blood. "Purification of the blood" may sound to some people like a claim from a wild west medicine show, but it's quite possible to help the blood cleanse itself of toxic wastes ... indeed that's what artificial kidneys do, in fact, for people whose kidneys are unable to filter out toxic wastes that would otherwise kill them. Spring tonics and blood cleansing plant remedies are a traditional way of getting at skin conditions like eczema and furunculosis, for these conditions are often caused by substances that come from under the skin, and not always from outside "dirt." In some cases of deficiency diseases and abnormally lowered resistance, a skin condition may well be caused by the *absence* of some substance under the skin, and in such cases, too, plants may be of some help.

Eczema, for example, has been alleviated by a combination of internal plus external use of pansy like this: 1 cup of pansy tea every morning and 1 cup every evening for several weeks. Pour 1 cup of boiling water over 2 teaspoonful of crushed dried foliage (that is, the above-ground parts), steep 5 minutes, strain, and drink. Then dip cotton pledgets or sterile gauze pads into the same pansy foliage tea and apply them to chronic eczema several times a day for same-day relief while the tea you drank develops its effect over several weeks. The powdered dried plant, too, has been sprinkled into wounds. Avoid long-term uninterrupted use of pansy, though, for too much of it might irritate the skin instead of healing it.

A traveling fertilizer salesman was suffering from an eczema which came from one or both of two possible causes: either the strong fertilizers and herbicides he lugged in his car, or else the emotional strain of trying to convince some headstrong farmers to stop using their natural manures and latrine slush so they could buy his synthetic products. In either case, his physician wanted to prescribe some pansy tea, but the salesman didn't care to stop and brew tea along the way. So, some of the time, he carried a thermos bottle with his day's pansy tea in it (just like Chinese hospital pharmacies send the day's teas up on the wards); other days he carried a finely crushed powder made from dried pansy foliage, and,

3 times a day, put half a teaspoonful of it in a cup of hot water, sweetened it with a little honey, and drank it for on-the-road blood purification, that is, for caring for his eczema from the inside out.

How a cattle raiser dissolved his stomach stones with a protein-digesting breakfast food that also dissolves warts and cleans up carious tooth pulp

The papaya "tree" (*Carica papaya*) is a giant shrub that can grow as high as 25 or 30 feet. Its melon is a common breakfast and dessert food. Papain, one of the enzymes in the papaya's milky sap, is often called a *vegetable pepsin* because it's similar to the enzyme pepsin, in our digestive system. But the papaya pepsin, unlike our animal pepsin, can act whether its surroundings are acid, alkaline, or neutral. Dental surgeons have used it to dissolve dead tissues down in the root canals of decayed teeth, and surgeons have applied it to dissolve infected tissues. Native peoples in tropical America have long known how to tenderize meat by rubbing it with the papaya's milky sap, or leaving it wrapped up several hours in papaya leaves. A Kansas stockman hit upon the idea of mixing a papain-containing tenderizer with milk or juice and drinking it to dissolve his gastric bezoars (stomach stones). Some people may react allergically to various parts of the fresh papaya plant, mainly, probably, the sap; in many cases, however, "allergies" to various plants turned out to be reactions only to herbicides and pesticides on the plants, not the plants themselves. Besides enzymes, papaya also contains alkaloids saponins, and at least 212 amino acids.

A fruit whose foliage and flowers are sedative, anti-spasmodic, anti-neuralgic and lower the blood pressure

The passion flower or may pop plant (*Passiflora incarnata*), whose fruit makes delicious eating, mildly sedates the nerves and overcomes insomnia, and helps relieve neuralgic aches and spasmodic asthma. There is uncertainty as to the substance(s) responsible for the sedative effect, but we do know that passion flower contains flavonoids, an alkaloid, and a substance that lowers the blood pressure. Aside from its fruit (the tasty "wild apricot" of the Cherokee Indians), it's best to use the other parts of passion flower and concentrated extracts only in professionally prepared remedies.

How a dock worker relieved his rope and charcoal burns with a mineral-laden fruit that also discourages uric acid stones

The pear (*Pyrus communis*) may be named from the Latin word for *fire,* referring to the flame shape of the fruit. Pear juice, a good source of minerals, reportedly breaks up uric acid compounds so as to prevent the formation of uric acid stones in the urinary passages. Pear leaf tea fights urinary infections, a property explained by the presence of the phenolglycoside arbutin (a urinary antiseptic) in the leaves.

For relieving his minor burns he got from the charcoal hibachi on which he cooked, and from rope burns, a Singapore dock worker crushed fresh pear seeds and plastered them over his burns.

The spice a pharmacist used to relieve his coughing and sciatica

Our word pepper is from the Greek word for pepper, *peperi,* or from *pepto* (meaning *to digest*) because pepper certainly helps digestion. Pepper has, in fact, been called a "fat digester." Both black and white peppers are from the same plant. Black pepper (*Piper nigrum*) is unripened and unhusked pepper fruits; white pepper (*Piper album*) is ripened and husked pepper fruits. And ground black pepper is a mixture of the black outside and whitish inside ... that's why you can see whitish specks mixed in with the black of peppercorns after you grind them.

The ancients were aware of the value of pepper for preserving food and making it tasty, even if the food had already started to rot, which was not rare in the days of month-long uncooled shipments. The Gothic king Alaric demanded 3,000 pounds of pepper along with 5,000 pounds of gold and 10,000 pounds of silver as ransom for the city of Rome when he laid siege to it in 408 A.D.

Pepper contains ethereal oil, the alkaloid piperin that gives pepper its sharp taste, and other substances. Paprika, a pepper or capsicum (*Capsicum annuum* and other species) of great importance to Hungarian paprikash cookery, supplies quite a load of vitamin C—more, in fact, than we obtain from oranges, grapefruit and lemons. In one set of tests, 100 grams of paprika contained about 107 milligrams of vitamin C, but 100 grams of orange, lemon or grapefruit contained only 30 to 36 milligrams of that vitamin. West German authorities, as a matter of fact, recently suggested that citizens there protect themselves from winter colds by eating more paprika. There are, by the way, sweet as well as sharp or hot varieties, so even though you don't like real peppery foods, you can still enjoy the milder sorts of paprikash dishes.

For his sciatic pains, a Macao pharmacist boiled up a rubbing lotion from long pepper (*Piper longum*), mustard oil, ginger root, and buttermilk curds. For bronchitic coughs, he drank (now and then during the course of the day) ½ to 2 ounces of a tea he made by boiling 2 ounces of powdered long pepper in 40 ounces of water until only 20 ounces of water remained in the porcelain crucible he always used (instead of metal) for compounding herbal remedies. Sips of this tea eased his coughing bouts in a few moments, and gave him relief for 1 to 4 hours.

A candy-flavoring plant that aids digestion and dispels headaches

The *pepper* part of peppermint (*Mentha piperita*) comes from the pepper-like or pungent taste of the plant. The *mint* part comes from the Greek nymph *Minthe*, whom the jealous queen of the underworld changed into a plant. Like pepper, peppermint helps digestion, especially gallbladder function . When I was a student at a German university and ordered a cup of tea in a nearby village inn, the innkeeper asked me whether I wanted black tea or peppermint tea. He said students often ate unwisely and studied too hard, so that's why he thought I wanted peppermint tea for my stomach. Peppermint (especially as an unsweetened tea) relieves gas, nausea, diarrhea, and griping cramps. It also combats inflammation in the intestinal tract, particularly of the gallbladder and bile ducts. It also stimulates healthy heart and nerve function. Besides menthol-containing ethereal oil, peppermint also contains tannins, bitters, and various other substances which account for its usefulness.

Several cups of peppermint leaf tea daily help overcome digestive distress, but don't drink it more than a week or so at a time without interruption. If your digestive distress continues, then perhaps you'd better review your diet, retrain your cook, take a hard look at your mealtime habits (do you argue or discuss business at the table?), or even consult a physician.

Peppermint oil, available at some druggists and food stores that stock genuine (not synthetic or artificial) spices and flavorings, has been rubbed on painful rheumatic and neuralgic spots, as well as on bruises.

Peppermint leaf tea (prepared as usual by pouring 1 cup of boiling water over a 1 teaspoonful or so of crushed dried leaves, and steeped 5 minutes before straining out the plant parts) helps against phlegm, coughs, gas, and stomach cramps when several cups a day are drunk, but not longer than for about 2 weeks at any one time without a break, for too much of it could irritate the gastrointestinal tract.

An aged rural Adirondacks doctor told me how he cured his lady patients of most of their headaches by soaking a folded washcloth in a cupful of cool water to which he added 1 teaspoonful of peppermint oil or essence, then laying the cloth over the forehead and temples of the patient.

A management analyst who worked for a computer firm suffered from spastic colon, for which he could find no relief even after consulting various physicians for over a year. Finally, in Arizona, he met an old lady, an Indian herbalist (sounds trite, but it's true) who at first suggested camomile tea (which didn't help too much), then peppermint and linden tea ... which at long last did work. The relief, however, did require a little patience, for he had to drink 1 cupful a day for 6 days a week for a month before pain and tenderness subsided. When a few twinges of pain and discomfort still occurred (after a particularly harassing day of racing back and forth to keep up with computer-induced frustration, which made him jumpy, or after too long a jog), the analyst told me, the discomfort was hardly noticeable, compared with how it affected him when he didn't drink the tea; at the time of this writing, he's been drinking the tea for a year and a half.

A zinc-storing antibacterial, anti-bleeding and cough-soothing leaf

Mucilage-rich plantain (*Plantago lanceolata* or lance-leaf plantain, and *Plantago major* or broad-leaf plantain) foliage and leaves soothe throat and bronchial irritations, including coughing and hoarseness. If plantain grows on zinc-rich soil, it stores up this important trace element, thus making a good dietary source of zinc. Zinc activates insulin and participates in ridding the body of carbon dioxide. Zinc deficiency is associated with a reduced sense of taste and slower healing of wounds.

Fresh plantain juice is antibacterial and helps stop bleeding, thus promoting the healing of wounds, boils and irritated, bleeding hemorrhoids. Toothache has been relieved temporarily by chewing on a piece of rootstock from the broad-leaved plantain.

Besides mucilage, plantain also contains enzymes, silicon compounds, vitamin C (ascorbic acid), alkaloids, tannin, xanthophyll (a yellow pigment described in the section on stinging nettle), and other substances. This plantain, by the way, is not related to the banana-like tropical plantain which figures so deliciously in Latin-American and other cookery.

A recipe for plantain tea is to pour a cupful of boiling water over 3 teaspoonsful of crushed dried lance-leaf leaves and steep 10 minutes before straining out the leaf fragments.

What pollen grains do for physical performance

Mighty oaks grow not only from tiny acorns, but even from much tinier pollen grains, so small that you need a microscope to see them, except for the giant ones that look like dust to the naked eye. These microscopic packages of vital energy have long been helping Eastern European athletes achieve their peak form and performance at international events. Pollen also helped Polish soldiers adapt quickly to the stress of being airlifted to a radically different climate—the desert around the Suez Canal and the Sinai peninsula—by the United Nations to help monitor the Mideast peace. Tests made among these Polish troops showed that daily dosage of fermented flower pollen (cernitin), especially with hydrolyzed protein (protein molecules broken down by the action of water), could increase the soldiers' capacity for effort and could shorten the time needed to reach peak form in the new environment. Pollen helped them to adapt to the desert faster by stepping up tolerance to new climatic conditions and by reinforcing the body's general resistance. The soldiers who did not take either the pollen or the protein never regained their initial fitness until they left the Middle East. These effects of pollen on the body and its functions are believed due to the combination of the cernitin with hydrolyzed protein, developed in Sweden.

Poland is not the only iron-curtain (or eastern block) country to make use of pollen to increase or improve physical fitness. Here is an excerpt from a letter written by the Light Athletics Federation of the USSR (Moscow) to a Swedish producer of pollen and protein extracts:

> The preparations which we received from you have been used in the training of Soviet light athletes for very demanding competitions... the products Stark protein, Pollitabs Sport and Cernitol improve sports performance ... and provide active relief from stress and strain ... the products do not have any harmful side effects ... they increase sportsmen's resistance to unfavorable factors. ...

> Yours very truly,

> Dr. A.V (Physician of the Light Athletics Federation of the USSR) and N.E.P ____ (Chief Trainer of the Light Athletics Sports Theme in the USSR)

Natural "aspirin" trees for reducing uric acid and alleviating arthritis, neuralgia rheumatism, hemorrhoids, and fever

The black poplar or aspen (*Populus nigra*) leaf buds, collected in winter while they are still closed, then air dried, contain salicin and populin, two phenolglycosides that combine into salipopulin, a natural compound that reduces the amount of uric acid in the blood, leading to excretion of the uric acid in the urine. This natural action, which doesn't put any stress on the kidneys or irritate them, contributes to the treatment program for alleviating chronic polyarthritis—a disease involving excess uric acid in the body. The salicin accounts for the pain-relieving effect on rheumatic joints and muscles.

Salicin also comes from willow trees and other plants that provided a natural aspirin for reducing pain and fever long before we knew how to industrially make aspirin from salicylic acid—a substance that's formed, by the way, when salicin-containing plant remedies pass through the body.

The tannin, flavonoids, ethereal oil, and other substances in poplar buds account for their other favorable effects, such as promoting the healing of wounds and relieving painfully swollen hemorrhoids.

The closed, winter leaf buds of *Populus gileadensis,* called balm of Gilead buds, are also a remedy, and may be the same as the "balm of Gilead" mentioned in this Negro spiritual:

> There is a balm in Gilead to make the wounded whole
> There is a balm in Gilead to heal the sin-sick soul

Some scholars, however, say that the balm of Gilead in that spiritual may not be of the poplar tree, but the balm of Gilead mentioned in Genesis and Jeremiah, a different plant.

Powdered bark of the white poplar or quaking aspen (*Populus tremuloides*), as well as of the black poplar, has been used for indigestion, fever, and as a tonic.

Willow (*Salix alba*) was around in Old England as *wilowe,* and even before that as Anglo-Saxon *welig* and old German *wida.* The willow tree symbolizes immortality in China, Iran, and elsewhere, accounting no doubt for its being planted in cemeteries. Willow inner bark tea is the original aspirin—it cools down fevers and alleviates rheumatic, neuralgic, and arthritic pains. Willow can also act antiseptically along the urinary passages and the gastrointestinal tract. The substances in willow responsible for these effects include tannins and glycosides (especially salicin).

A Belgrade doctor whose rural experience stood him in good stead during periods of wartime shortages made willow tea to sip during the day when an aspirin-like effect was needed, by soaking a small handful (or several large pinches) of willow inner bark (stripped from the trees in springtime) for about 3 hours in 1 cup of cold water, then quickly brought it to a boil, removed it from the heat and strained out the bark before use.

A midwestern trapper extracted salicin from poplar and willow trees for use as a pain-killer for his headaches and rheumatic aches. He poured boiling water over willow leaves and female flowers, or over powdered willow or poplar inner bark strips, then steeped it about 10 minutes before straining out the bark. A cup or two of the tea gave him the same benefit as a few aspirin.

An American Indian "aspirin" shrub that alleviated a bargeman's headachy weather woes

Wintergreen, Canada tea, or mountain tea (*Gaultheria procumbens*) was an American Indian remedy utilized by a Dr. Gautier of Quebec, hence the scientific name *Gaultheria*. A similar species of wintergreen was used by the British in India, too, where they put a few drops of it into their inkpots to protect against the everpresent problem of mold growth. Mildly pain-relieving wintergreen liniment, like willow bark, relieves rheumatic and arthritic pains, neuralgia around the ribs, and sciatica.

A Great Lakes bargeman eased his wet-weather woes and headachy feeling by sipping a cup or so a day of wintergreen tea he brewed by pouring 1 cupful of boiling water over 1 teaspoonful of autumn wintergreen leaves.

The aromatic, aspirin-like methyl salicylate from the ethereal oil in wintergreen leaves not only largely accounts for these properties and effects, but can also free victims from various tiny creatures that infest their skin and hair

A farmer's plow-stopping root that aids victims of gout and urinary stones

The deep roots of restharrow or stayplough (*Ononis spinosa*) certainly bring the farmer's plow (or plough) to rest The German name *Harnkraut* for this root reveals its use to promote good urinary flow, especially of the chlorine and urea components of the body's waste fluids. This property accounts in part for its use in relieving gout by helping to flush out the substances that form uric acid, crystals of which accumulate in the joints of gout victims or form urinary stones. Restharrow's effects are due to its ethereal oil, flavonoids, tannin, and other constituents.

Some Europeans who use this plant to ease their gout, drink about 2 or 3 cups of the root tea a day, while others drink only half a cupful. One way they make the tea is by soaking 1 tablespoonful of chopped dried root in half a cupful of cold water overnight, heating to the boiling point, then letting it cool down a bit before drinking. Another way they brew the tea is by pouring 1 cupful of boiling water over a small handful of root chips and steeping it for 5 to 10 minutes before straining out the chips.

A vegetable dessert that moves the bowels but also stops diarrhea

Rhubarb (*Rheum* species) illustrates the need for guidance when going afield to "benefit from nature's storehouse" of useful plants. We all know that the pinkish, celery-like rhubarb leaf stalks are a common dessert food, but when we decide to use even more of a good thing by eating rhubarb leaves as well as the leaf stalks, we run into trouble. The leaf blades contain tiny, sharp crystals of calcium and potassium oxalates. Under some conditions and in some people, these crystals can severely irritate the throat. Just the stalks should be used. Small amounts of rhubarb aid digestion and control diarrhea, but larger amounts are laxative.

Rhubarb contains anthraquinones, tannins, flavonoids (such as rutin), resin, pectin, and other substances.

How a vitamin-rich fruit helped a trucker's disrupted digestion

Dog rose (*Rosa canina*) "fruit" is only pseudofruit which contains the real fruit ... which looks like the seeds, and this seed-like fruit encloses the actual seeds. All of that botanical precision, however, would be too disconcerting if we carried it too far, for then we'd have to admit that even our strawberries are merely the imbedding mass for the real fruit—those tiny little grains which give the strawberries their characteristic surface texture. The old English word *hips* for rose fruit remains with us today.

Rose hips contain vitamins (C, A, B1, B2, K, nicotinic acid or niacin, P or rutin, and E) as well as tannin, fruit sugars, ethereal oil, flavonoids, pectin, and other substances. All of these make rose hips not only a valuable vitamin supplement, but also give them the power to alleviate enteritis, gallstones, and stones in the urinary tract.

A Hungarian trucker who often ate irregularly during his international long-hauls, brewed rose hip tea for his digestion by boiling a large pinch of ground-up "seeds" (that is, the real seed-containing structures within the fleshy pseudofruit) in 1 cupful of cold water until only half the cupful of water remained, which he sipped during the day. Sometimes his wife mashed up the pseudofruit and brewed an ordinary breakfast tea by pouring boiling water over it.

Although heat destroys vitamin C, a fast application of high heat (like a quick dousing with boiling water) destroys less of it than does a slow application of low heat. This is true for rose hips or other vitamin C-rich foodstuffs. According to one study, the drying process may destroy 45% to 90% of the vitamin C in rose hips.

Two other ways to brew rose hip tea are (1) Soak 2 teaspoonsful of crushed "seeds" or apparent pits for 5 to 7 hours in 1 cup of cold water, then bring to a quick boil before drinking the tea either warm or cold. (2) Boil 2 teaspoonsful of crushed "seeds" for 10 minutes, steep 10 minutes, and strain out the plant parts before drinking.

The herb a waitress used for menstrual regularity and clearing up discharges

Rosemary (*Rosmarinus officinalis*) leaves' ethereal oil, tannin, niacin, saponin, and flavonoids promote the healing of wounds, aid digestion, and, as an ointment or liniment, ease the pains of rheumatism, arthritis, and neuritis.

For low blood pressure (also, bruises, rheumatism, varicose veins), a tonic rosemary bath can be prepared by pouring 1 pint of boiling water over 50 grams of rosemary leaves, steeping about 5 minutes, then adding this tea or infusion to your bathwater for a 10-minute bath at body temperature (98° to 99° F), followed by 30 minutes of bed rest, as recommended by European physicians who prescribe this tonic bath for their patients. Because this rosemary bath tones you up and improves circulation (instead of calming you down like, say, a valerian bath), it is taken in the afternoon or in the morning, but not just before bed, for you'd be too toned up to sleep well.

An Austrian waitress drank rosemary tea (1 cupful of boiling water poured over 1 teaspoonful of crushed leaves, and steeped for 5 minutes) for keeping her menstrual periods regular. She also used the rosemary tea as a douche to clear up her vaginal discharge (leukorrhea). Several douches a day helped control the discharge and ease irritation for several hours. Another way to make rosemary tea is to bring 1 teaspoonful of crushed dried leaves in 1 cupful of cold water to a boil (in a coated or non-metallic pot), and then strain out the leaves. (Boiling tends to drive away more of a plant's ethereal oil, but draws more tannins and other non-volatile substances out of the plant parts and into the water.

Cervantes, the creator of the classic Spanish tale of Don Quijote—that chivalrous old gentleman who went about saving damsels in distress and attacking windmills—had his characters caring for their wounds by washing them with an old Spanish recipe of rosemary, olive oil, wine, and salt.

A vitamin C-rich tree whose fruit can help glaucoma victims and diabetics

The rowan or roan or European mountain ash tree (*Sorbus aucuparia*) berries are rich in vitamin C, and the sorbose or sorbit sugar in the fruit can replace the glycerine often taken by glaucoma sufferers to reduce pressure in their eyes. This sugar is also a safe substitute for diabetics.

The berries promote the flow of urine and act mildly laxative, but can also stop diarrhea if they are first cooked to destroy the laxative substance, thus letting the tannin and pectin act. This ash tree also contains fruit acids, carotinoids, bitters, phenolglycoside, and other substances.

Rowan leaves have been brewed for a refreshing tea; the flowers brewed for a mild laxative; the bark boiled for an anti-diarrheal tea.

A hernia-relieving plant

Rupturewort (*Herniaria glabra* or *Hernaria hirsuta*) foliage tea was once thought to cure hernia or rupture, but its real effect was apparently only to relieve painfully cramped urinary passages by relaxing or widening them, thus alleviating discomfort ... which indeed was some help if not a cure. Rupturewort—which has also been used by rural folk for easing the discomfort of cystitis, urethritis, and old cases of syphilis—contains flavonoids, saponins, tannin, ethereal oil, inulin, and perhaps an alkaloid.

Rupturewort foliage tea is brewed in the usual way by pouring boiling water over crushed dried foliage and steeping awhile.

The spice a salesman gargled for laryngitis, an asthmatic inhaled to breathe easier, and a computer operator used to relieve eyestrain

Sage's scientific name *Salvia* is from Latin *salvus* for *saved* not only because it saves the user from health problems, but also because it preserved the edibility of meat before the era of refrigeration. Sage inhibits sweating (especially night sweats) and lactation in nursing mothers, lowers the amount of sugar in the blood of diabetics, relieves gastrointestinal cramping and gas, and acts antiseptically to reduce mouth and throat infections as well as to alleviate chronic bronchial inflammation.

Sage contains ethereal oil, tannins, saponin, bitters, an estrogen-like substance that normalizes menstruation, resin, flavonoids, and an anti-tubercular bacillus substance.

To soothe his sore throat and laryngitis, and ease his wife's toothache, a Berlin salesman prepared a sage tea and gargle in the usual manner, that is, he poured 1 cupful of boiling water over 1 teaspoonful of crushed sage leaves and steeped it for 5 minutes.

To ease his bronchial distress, an Idaho asthmatic inhaled the smoke from dried sage leaves which he ignited either in an ashtray, or rolled into cigarette paper and smoked like a cigarette. Inhalation of the smoke suppressed much of his bronchial distress during mild bouts. When he went out camping or on picnics, he rubbed crushed fresh sage leaves on any insect stings his family suffered, and relief was immediate. He also applied sage leaves to poorly healing sores to hasten healing.

A Venezuelan woman whose eyes became reddened and watery from too many hours of entering data on the screen of a computer terminal in a windowless room, couldn't find an ophthalmologist in Miami capable of relieving her eye discomfort. Finally, a Cuban friend brewed her a sage eyewash from fresh sage leaves (brewed like the tea described above) and the eye inflammation cleared up by the next day after two eyebaths (from an eyecup) during the day, followed by 15 minutes with a compress of warmed sage tea over her eyes just before bed.

A digestion-promoting thistle that helped a pharmacist recuperate and protect herself from bronchitis

Saint Benedict's thistle or blessed thistle or holy thistle or cardin (*Cnicus benedictus* or *Centaurea benedicta*) foliage and "seeds" (really fruit) aid digestion by stimulating bile and gastric juices, just as other plants that contain bitters do. Besides bitters, Saint Benedict's thistle also contains mucilage, tannins, a little ethereal oil, flavonoids, resins, and niacin. These and other substances contribute to the other properties of this thistle, which include getting phlegm up, acting antimicrobially, and fighting fevers.

Large amounts of this plant might nauseate. Expectant mothers should have a physician's approval before using it, a good general caution for any pregnant women who take any substances or expose themselves to any unaccustomed activity.

A Polish pharmacist helped her own recovery and lack of appetite, and protected herself from recurrence of bronchitis and fever by drinking 1 cupful of Saint Benedict's "seed" tea (1 teaspoonful of crushed "seeds" boiled in cup of water) a day. Her father sipped a tea (1 tablespoon of "seed" boiled in about 1 pint of water) during the day to ease his gas, biliary, and liver problems.

How a red-dotted yellow-flowered plant that heals wounds dried up a bed wetter and lifted menopausal depression

The yellow petals of Saint John's wort (*Hypericum perforatum*) are dotted with dark spots that at first glance look like perforations. Legend has it that these spots turn blood-red on August 29th, the day John the Baptist was beheaded. In fact, a purple-red color does appear if you squeeze the flower petals.

Although scientists are not quite decided as to *how* Saint John's wort acts sedatively and helps sufferers of nervous system conditions (such as neuralgia, insomnia, depression, menopausal neurosis, bedwetting, and brain concussion), the scientists have indeed verified that it does help. Also, Saint John's wort is used to control diarrhea, to heal wounds and burns, and, in general, to reduce inflammation.

Saint John's wort contains ethereal oil, flavonoids (including rutin), tannins, pigment, niacin, pectin and hypericin—a substance which promotes circulation in the capillaries, and which may be responsible for the plant's favorable effect on mental conditions. Overuse of the plant, by the way, can temporarily photosensitize some people, that is, make them temporarily oversensitive to sunlight, predisposing them to sunburn.

Saint John's wort has been used in the form of a juice from the whole plant, as a tea, and as an oily liniment prepared commercially.

A North Dakota man helped his son to stop wetting his bed by giving him a cup of Saint John's wort tea (1 cupful of boiling water poured over 1 teaspoonful of crushed dried foliage, and steeped 10 minutes) an hour or so before bed ... but the man always left his son an hour or so of time between drinking and sleeping to empty his bladder before bed! Another recipe to control bedwetting is to sip, throughout the day, 2 to 3 cups of cooled, unsweetened Saint John's wort tea prepared by boiling 1 tablespoonful of foliage in 1 cupful of water for 2 minutes.

To be sure they have the right species or variety of Saint John's wort, Alpine herbalists crush the half-opened flower to see if a blood-red juice oozes out; if so, it's the right plant.

A woman from Cologne, Germany, was advised by her physician to drink Saint John's wort tea to help her overcome menopausal depression. She drank 1 cup of the tea warm at breakfast and 1 cup in the evening, continuing this pattern for several weeks. To prepare the tea, she poured 1 cupful of boiling water over 1 tablespoonful of the crushed dried foliage, steeped it 5 minutes, then strained out the plant parts before she drank it' When she took this course of tea-drinking during the summer, she avoided excessive exposure to bright sunlight to eliminate the possibility of being predisposed to sunburn (since Saint John's wort can photosensitize in some cases).

A thistle that helped a bartender's liver ward off environmental toxins

The seed-like fruit of Saint Mary's thistle, milk thistle, holy thistle or marythistle (*Carduus marianus* or *Silybum marinum*) cools down fevers, protects liver cells and supports the liver in its work of neutralizing and/or eliminating the natural and unnatural poisons that pass through us daily, as well as those which we just happen to swallow now and then, like toadstool poisons. Saint Mary's thistle's apparent ability to protect membranes no doubt contributes to that detoxifying power. In addition, this thistle's seed-like fruit has alleviated swollen liver, "stitches" in the side, gallbladder colic, and seasickness. These effects are due to the plant's tannin, bitters, ethereal oil, flavonoids (including silymarin, a substance that protects the liver from toxins), mucilage (in the roots), resin, and amino acids.

The bartender of a large resort hotel suffered from generally poor stomach and digestive function as well as poor liver function, so he took the advice of one of his customers—a lady pharmacist from Basle, Switzerland—and swallowed a pinch of crushed Saint Mary's thistle seeds with a gulp of water at different times throughout the day. In a few days, his dyspepsia and upset stomach cleared up enough that he could feel the difference from his usual dyspeptic self. His appetite improved and he digested better whatever he now ate. (His food became less the soggy sandwiches he was in the habit of gulping down as he stood behind his bar, and became more the just as inexpensive yet more appetizing yoghurt, cheese, fresh vegetables, and fruit he began to eat slowly while sitting in a nearby park overlooking the ocean). In a week or so, he looked less jaundiced, that is, you could see that he had a healthier skin tone— at least you saw it whenever he stepped out of the subdued lighting of the hotel bar and lounge, and onto the sunny terrace!

A small palm whose sedative berries strengthen the genito-urinary organs

The saw palmetto, sabal, dwarf or scrub palm (*Serenoa serrulata*) of the eastern and southern part of North America, produces berries with nutritive and tonic properties, especially on our hormonal system. The first part of its scientific name, *Serenoa*, is in honor of the botanist who first described it, Sereno Watson. The second part, *serrulata* (meaning *little saw* in Latin) refers to the leaf stalk, which is armed with very sharp spines arranged saw-like along the edge. It's one of those coincidences that the botanist's first name, *Sereno*, is Spanish for *serene* or *calm*—physicians who prescribed the saw palmetto berries to build up strength in their patients who were victims of wasting diseases found that there was also a calming effect along with the fortifying effect of the berries.

Saw palmetto berries seem to preserve and strengthen organically healthy but tired or even functionally weak genito-urinary and other organs, especially hormonally controlled ones like the testes, mammary glands, and prostate.

Saw palmetto berries contain ethereal oil, fatty acids, flavonoids, carotene, enzymes, tannin, resin, estrogen-like substances, among other substances, all of which contribute not only to the plant's medicinal use, but also make it useful industrially to aromatize cognac.

A nutritious mucilage-rich
seaweed for soothing irritated
and inflamed tissues

Seaweeds, a common name for marine algae, are a link with our ancestral source of nutrients, the sea. In sea water, many minerals may be so dilute that we can't use them directly as food. We can, however, eat the mineral-laden seaweeds, which accumulate and concentrate in their cells the tiniest traces of minerals from the sea waters in which they grow—and they grow large indeed, such as the kelp fronds and stalks which have been reported to reach lengths of 100 to 300 feet. The unique contribution of seaweed to our health may well be this power to concentrate the minerals we need. Seaweeds also provide vitamins and certain polysaccharides found only in sea plants. Despite the fact that people who live from the sea have benefited from these virtues since the beginning of time, medicine today is just starting to discover the startling properties of these substances from the kingdom below the sea. The healthful properties of seaweed and other sea life are described in detail in *Helping Yourself to Health from the Sea*, Parker Publishing Co.

Irish moss or carrageen (*Chondrus crispus*) is a common seaweed which is quite useful as a nutritious dietary supplement for convalescents, and a soothing remedy for bronchitis, coughing and other conditions in which this seaweed's mucilaginous properties can ease chapped, raw skin and irritations, as well as inflammations such as cystitis and gastroenteritis. A tea is made by boiling 1 teaspoonful of the dried frond in 1 cupful of water, or 2 teaspoonsful of the seaweed can be boiled at once in 2 cups of water, thus making up the daily dosage of 1 to 2 cups taken by some Europeans for soothing irritated membranes.

An ancient Nubian yellow-flowered
plant to loosen the bowels

Senaar in ancient Nubia was one of the places where senna grew natively, hence the plant's name. Senaar is probably the present

Sennar in eastern Sudan between the Blue and the White Nile rivers, south of Khartoum. The laxative plant *senna* may actually be any of the following three species: (1) the leaves of American or wild senna (*Cassia marilandica*), (2) the leaves and pods of Alexandrian senna (*Cassia* or *Senna acutifolia*), or (3) the leaves of Tinnevelly senna (*Cassia angustifolia*).

People who take senna leaves or pods for their laxative effect are sometimes surprised, if not thrown into complete panic, when they pass carmine-red urine! But this happens only if their urine happens to be alkaline at the time they take senna. A Swiss pharmacist told me that the senna leaf teas also stimulate normal menstruation.

Senna contains emodine anthraquinines, flavonoids, ethereal oil, resin, and other substances. Don't boil remedies that contain senna, for the intense heat can change some of these ingredients into compounds that might cause stomach pain or griping.

A British pharmacologist suggested brewing tea from the leaves of American or wild senna in the usual way (pouring 1 cupful of boiling water over about 1 teaspoonful of plant material) but steeping it somewhat longer than usual, that is, steep it 20 to 30 minutes. Or, he suggested, soak 3 to 6 Alexandrian pods in 150 milliliters of warm water for 6 to 12 hours. This British pharmacologist also suggested the addition of crushed cardamom, fennel, or ginger root before pouring the water over the senna; these spices keep the senna from causing griping while it goes about moving your bowels. Users of senna are cautioned not to take it if they have gastrointestinal inflammations (including hemorrhoids).

An oil plant for easing bowel movements and promoting healthy hair growth. A natural-foaming oil for skin and stomach. A salad-oil flower that helps malaria victims, stops bleeding, and makes a non-junk-food snack for thousands of sport fans

Sesame seed (*Sesamum indica*) was sold in the streets of Delhi by itinerant confectioners who sang this ditty to praise their wares:

Sesame, tikhur* and linseed
Butter and sugar, poppy seed
Old men it makes quite young with speed.

Besides its use as a pleasant carrier for other substances that dissolve in its oil, sesame was known in India for its nourishing and tonic properties, for its promotion of the flow of urine, and for easing bowel movement so as to relieve the pressure on painfully swollen hemorrhoids. Sesame was used in hairwashes to promote the growth and black sheen of hair. Also, it was used to relieve gallbladder distress. The Turkish candy *halvah*, too, is made of sesame. Sesame seeds contain fatty oil, protein, vitamins (B, D, E, F), lecithin, and other substances. The mucilage-rich leaves are still used as a tea in India to ease chronic dysentery.

Besides sesame, peanut, safflower and olive oils for healthy cuisine and salads, there's coconut nut oil, too, for natural cookery. I watched and hungrily smelled Central American Indians soak coconut meat in water out in the hot tropical sun all day until the coconut's oil rose to the surface, from where it was scooped off and used to fry freshly netted fish. Coconut oil is a natural foamer that's good for your skin as well as your stomach. The ecological advantage of coconut foam is that it's biodegradable, that is, after it carries out its function in your bath or whatever product it was part of, it can be broken down by natural means and dissipated in the flow of matter around us. Unlike some synthetic detergents that go on and on and on floating around and polluting the waterways, coconut oils go back into Mother Nature's never-ending mill of creation, transformation, and recreation.

As long as we're on the subject of oils, we can mention sunflower oil, a common kitchen item, pressed from a plant once used by Virginia Indians against intermittent fever—a use which led physicians to believe that extract of sunflower (*Helianthus annuus*) petals may help victims of malaria not treatable by other means. The flower also provides pectin to stop bleeding. Sunflower's numerous

---

*Indian curcuma or arrowroot

seeds, which yield a good salad oil, make a nutritious, non-junk-food snack for thousands of sport fans in some countries (like the Rumanian soccer fans, for example, who munch on them the way Americans chew on popcorn and chewing gum), and make a nourishing addition to bread flours—and also a fine bird seed. Besides its oils, sunflower contains xanthophyll, lecithin, tannin, amino acids, flavonoids, and other substances.

A white-flowered vascular-active, muscle-relaxing, sedative, antimicrobial, and anti-fertility plant

The seed pods of shepherd's purse or poor man's pharmacy (*Capsella bursa-pastoris*) are rather skimpy like a flattened, poorly filled shepherd's purse, hence one of its names. Its other name, *poor man's pharmacy*, reflects its frequent use as a home remedy. It's been used to stop bleeding, particularly of the uterus, but also of hemorrhoids, the lungs, and other organs. Heart-toning, muscle-relaxing, sedative, antimicrobial, anti-fertility and vascular-active effects have been reported for this plant. Although the vessel-tightening effect of the plant helps explain how it controls bleeding and how it raises blood pressure, it doesn't account for the reportedly hypotensive (or anti-hypertensive) effect which helps to keep blood pressure within normal limits—that is, the plant has been reported not only to raise blood pressure, but also to lower it, this dual effect having led to shepherd's purse's use to regularize blood pressure, whichever way (up or down) it needs to go to keep normal. In any case, research is still underway on this and many other plants whose use is beneficial—but still unexplained. We do know that shepherd's purse contains flavonoids (including one with known anti-hemorrhagic effect), mustard oil, some tannin, ethereal oil, vitamin C, alkaloids, and other substances.

One European recipe for using this plant (2 cups a day, perhaps sweetened with some honey) is to boil 1 teaspoonful of foliage for 2 minutes in 1 cup of water. Another recipe is to pour 1 cup of boiling water over 1 teaspoonful to 1 tablespoonful of foliage, and steeping it 5 to 10 minutes before straining out the plant parts. Yet another recipe is to soak 1 to 2 tablespoonsful of the foliage in 1 cupful of cool water for about 8 hours.

A yellow flower that eased a tourist guide's menstrual and a French chef's gallbladder cramping

Silverweed (*Potentilla anserina*) gets its English name from the satiny-silvery undersides of its leaves. A cramp-reducing substance in silverweed explains another of its names, *crampweed*. Flavonoids and tannins, too, help account for many of the plant's effects.

For relief of menstrual distress, a Swedish tourist guide drank 2 or 3 cups daily of warm silverweed tea made by pouring 1 cupful of boiling water over 1 to 3 teaspoonsful of crushed dried foliage and then steeping 10 to 15 minutes before straining out the foliage. She drank the tea a few days before, and then during her actual period. From time to time she mixed up combinations of silverweed with camomile flowers, lemon balm (melissa) leaves, milfoil foliage, or valerian root for reinforcing the effect. (Many plants give better, that is, more effective, faster, more pleasant results when combined with other plants. The combination remedies later in this book are described for that reason.)

A Swiss herbalist said that 1 or 2 cups of silverweed tea drunk on 3 or 4 days a month can ward off strokes in people who are predisposed to them. He suggested for this purpose a tea somewhat weaker than the one described above, that is, he suggesed 1 teaspoonful per cup of water.

When a spoonful of good olive oil didn't ease his gallbladder cramping, a French chef in a Marseille restaurant found relief with a daily cup of silverweed tea (prepared as above) during his bouts of gallbladder problems.

Father Sebastian Kneipp—the 19th century "water doctor" who achieved so many therapeutic successes with simple, safe and natural means—found that silverweed or crampweed milk (1 tablespoonful of crushed leaves boiled in half a pint of milk) alleviated abdominal cramps—the remedy worked whether it was drunk or applied as a warm (or sometimes cool) compress on the skin just over the cramping. (Quite aside from the effect of the temperature of the compress, don't forget that many substances pass easily through the skin; the permeability of the skin to drugs and plant ingredients is the basis of quite a few thoroughly scientific treatments carried out by physicians and surgeons.)

Salad greens that eased an ex-shepherd's gallstone distress and kept a merchant's hair healthy

The stinging nettle (*Urtica dioica*) promotes excretion of chlorine and urea in the urine and slightly reduces the amount of sugar in the blood. Sufferers of rheumatism have even flogged themselves with stinging nettle foliage to provide immediate relief by counter-irritation! This flogging course of therapy may run once a day 2 to 3 days at a time. Less violently inclined gout and rheumatism victims have poured 2 cups of boiling water over 3 to 4 teaspoons of crushed leaves, steeped it 10 minutes and strained out the leaves before sipping the tea through the day. Others have made a stronger tea by using 3 tablespoonsful of the foliage and/or leaves per cup. The tea, of course, doesn't act as rapidly as the flogging, but does wash out the substances which tend to cause gout.

Tender young nettle leaves, without stinging hairs yet, and young plants which can be boiled to quell the hairs, make a fine salad vegetable which is rich in vitamin C, iron, chlorophyll, and xanthophyll.

Chlorophyll, the green pigment of plants, promotes the healing of ulcers, wounds, and burns, and also reduces unpleasant odors such as bad breath and certain malodorous conditions of the nose. In addition, chlorophyll stimulates metabolic processes, increases the number of thrombocytes and leukocytes in sufferers of anemia, protects against arteriosclerosis, and inhibits the growth of fungi.

Xanthophyll, which makes buttercups and other flowers yellow, is, unlike chlorophyll, not broken down in the digestive tract, but gets through to various organs where it works with hormones and vitamins to the benefit of the body. Xanthophyll favorably affects blood formation, enhances the growth effect of vitamin A, and, like chlorophyll, fosters the healing of wounds.

Stinging nettle owes it value not only to these green and yellow pigments, iron, and vitamin C, but also to its tannin, calcium, vitamin B2, pantothenic acid, glucokinine (an insulin-like hormone also found in onions and other plants), amino acids, and other substances, all of which really make up for its minor inconvenience—its stinging hairs.

A former Alpine shepherd showed me how he boiled stinging nettle leaves and roots in milk, and drank it to flush out more urine and ease his gallstone distress, which he began to suffer long after he gave up his shepherd's work and began to work in a large industrial city. He also stressed that although he enjoyed young, springtime stinging nettle foliage as a salad, he was always sure to boil or otherwise cook well any older, stinging nettle foliage before eating it; otherwise, he said, the hairs could irritate the kidneys.

For his hair care, an Italian merchant in Macao stocked up on a lotion he made by boiling fresh stinging nettle foliage (a handful or two, but with gloves!) in half a pint of vinegar (in a non-metallic pot) for 15 minutes, straining out the debris, and pouring it into well-stoppered bottles. He assured me that this lotion nourished his scalp and made him feel like his hair was growing stronger than ever—which could certainly have been true, judging from the looks of his head of thick, bushy hair.

A vitamin and mineral-charged fruit plant used in vein and wound remedies, and also enjoyed for breakfast by a businessman to ease his rheumatism and gout

Tea brewed from strawberry (*Fragaria vesca*) leaves makes a refreshing replacement for ordinary black (Chinese or Ceylonese or Javanese or Japanese) tea, and stops diarrhea, too, because the tannins in strawberry leaves act astringently on the tissues, that is, draws them together like a styptic pencil does to stem the blood that oozes out when you nick yourself shaving.

Rural folk use strawberries for alleviating gangrenous ulcers caused by frostbite, and strawberries are also employed in remedies for vein problems involving ulcers on the legs. The vitamin C in strawberries may be a reason for these uses, for vitamin C is used medically by physicians in the treatment of wounds and infections. The iron, phosphorus and other minerals in strawberries, too, contribute most definitely to the proper nutrition and functioning of the body. Strawberries also contain ethereal oil, flavonoids, pectin, and fruit acids.

A Munich professor, before the yearly hectic bustle of exams, drank a nerve tea brewed from strawberry leaves, thyme foliage, and woodruff or master of the wood (*Asperula odorata*) to gather himself together for a calm, quiet approach to his students.

An Austrian wine merchant advised me to eat fresh strawberries only *before* meals, and never to eat ice-cold strawberries if I wanted to avoid their disrupting my digestion. He was an expert on strawberries, for he not only sold strawberry wine and ate the fresh fruit regularly, but he also enjoyed strawberry leaf tea often to ease his rheumatism and gouty aches.

How a London Bobby alleviated respiratory distress with an insect-devouring plant that also removes warts and corns

The sundew (*Drosera rotundifolia*) sparkles with the early morning dew droplets that adhere to the stickly secretion on its tentacles—out to catch insects for its food. This insect-catching and insect-dissolving secretion contains an enzyme that breaks down protein, and no doubt contributes to this plant's reputed power to remove warts and corns. Sundew also contains plumbagin, a compound that acts antibiotically against disease-causing *Streptococcus, Staphylococcus, Pneumococcus* and probably also tuberculosis bacilli—all bad names when infections are involved. Besides the enzyme mentioned above, sundew also contains a little ethereal oil, tannin, resin, pigments, flavonoids, and other substances that account for its expectorant and cramp-relieving properties, and its use in alleviating coughs, bronchial asthma, and chronic bronchitis.

A London Bobby who was often on outside duty made a tea to ease his respiratory distress by pouring a cup of boiling water over half a teaspoonful (he didn't use too much because too much can irritate) of dried sundew foliage, steeped it about 5 minutes, and then sipped 1 to 2 cups of it a day. Sometimes he prepared his whole day's supply at once by pouring 2 cups of boiling water over a whole teaspoonful of the foliage.

An antiseptic and deodorant spice for respiratory, digestive, and skin health

Thyme (*Thymus vulgaris*) may be named after the *thym* plant which the ancient Egyptians used to prepare mummies. Thyme disinfects and deodorizes wounds, fights bacteria in the urinary passages, destroys intestinal worms, and may also be effective against hookworms. It controls nervous and dry cough, clears out phlegm, and helps respiratory passages irritated by inflammation and infection. Thyme promotes normal digestion by sparking appetite and relieving cramps, gas, and diarrhea. Rubbing with thyme liniment stops itching skin and alleviates underlying rheumatic pain.

A Swedish masseuse made a thyme bath for easing respiratory distress (caused by convulsive coughing and phlegm) by pouring 1 quart of boiling water over 100 grams of thyme foliage and steeping it for 5 minutes, then by adding that tea to her bathwater. Respiratory relief occurred within 10 minutes, when she began to breathe easier while still in her tub.

Thyme's phenol-rich ethereal oil, it has been shown, reaches a bather's troubled spots in two ways: (1) by absorption through the skin, and (2) by inhalation of the ethereal oil as it vaporizes from the surface of the bathwater. Thyme's tannin, bitters, resin, flavonoids, and a cramp-relieving substance contribute to its effects.

How a sea captain used spice to ease gallbladder distress

If you look on the label of the jar of mustard in your refrigerator, you'll see that one of the ingredients is tumeric (*Curcuma xanthorrhiza*, also called turmeric, curcuma, or Indian saffron)—a condiment that shows up in the curries of India—and has been in them since long before mustard was bottled or refrigerators were known. The label on the bottle of a popular brand of curry on my kitchen shelf lists seven spices (all of which are ground up into an orange powder): cumin, coriander, fenugreek, cardamom, red pepper, black pepper, and tumeric (which gives the powder its golden orange color).

The curcuma rhizome, prepared as a remedy, specifically relaxes cramping at the sphincter of Oddi.

A Dutch maritime captain eased his gallbladder distress by drinking 3 cups of tumeric rhizome tea daily. To make the tea, he added 1 tablespoonful of crushed rhizome to 1 cupful of cold water, brought it to a boil for a few minutes until he had enough yellow dye in the water, strained out the fragments of rhizome, and when it cooled down, drank it.

Don't confuse tumeric (also called *Indian* saffron) with Spanish or French saffron, which is from the stigmas of the flower *Crocus sativus*, the autumn crocus. A single drop of Spanish or French saffron will color 100,000 drops of water a distinct yellow—and although some estimates of Spanish or French saffron's toxicity run as high as 10 or 12 grams as a fatal dosage, others estimate that only a few grams can be fatal. The very tiny amounts of Spanish or French saffron used in cookery, however, should not cause any concern.

How an overwrought teacher allayed her nervous palpitations with a cat-attracting root that also soothes tired eyes

A caravan leader transporting bundles of valerian from Kabul in Afghanistan to Peshawar on the Kyber Pass once complained that "all the cats in the country surrounded me at night wherever we camped!" And that's why valerian (*Valeriana officinalis*) is also called *cat* valerian. It attracts them.

The name *valerian* comes from the Latin *valere* (meaning *to be strong*), referring to the medicinal value of the plant, known to the western world at least since a certain Izhak ben Soleiman mentioned it in his 9th or 10th century Latin translation of an Arabic medical treatise.

Valerian's virtues include an excellent sedative effect on the central nervous system, hence its use to induce rest and sleep, and, in general, to alleviate nervous excitability such as occurs with hysteria, migraine, rheumatism, and painful menstrual periods. Extracts of the plant also calm down nervousness and overly active reflexes in the gastrointestinal tract in such a way that colicky pains and cramping are alleviated. Valerian's sedative effects are believed due to its ethereal oil, but probably also to an alkaloid.

To soothe her tired eyes, a Swiss pharmacist applied valerian root tea with cotton balls or with an eyewash cup.

An aggravated Danish teacher who suffered from nervous palpitations at bedtime drank a cup of valerian tea before bed several times a week to ensure a good night's sleep. She soaked 1 teaspoonful of diced valerian root in a cupful of cold water all day, until, after dinner, she brought the water and root fragments to a boil, strained out the root pieces, and drank her tea. A herbalist in Copenhagen advised the teacher that if she drank 1 or 2 cups a day, that was quite enough, and that she shouldn't drink it continuously for more than a few weeks at any one time.

A garden ornamental plant for relieving respiratory inflammation and protecting against the spread of tumors

The saponins in violets (*Viola odorata*) account for their expectorant effect in breaking up and moving phlegm out of infected and inflamed respiratory passages. The salicylic acid in violets may also contribute to their soothing effect on painfully irritated tissues associated with colds and other respiratory conditions. Violets also contain odoratin (a substance that lowers blood pressure), ethereal oil, mucilage, and pigment.

Tea made from violet leaves, flowers, and/or rhizomes has been gargled to relieve sore throat and mouth, and difficulty in swallowing. One way to make such a tea is to soak 2 tablespoonsful of violet leaves, flowers, and root chips in 1 cupful of cold water for about 1½ hours, then bring it to a boil before removing from the heat and straining out the plant parts.

Various species of violet have shown anti-tumor effects in animals, and sweet violet (*Viola odorata*) is recommended in England to protect patients from metastasis (or spread of a growth to other parts of the body) after having their tumors surgically removed.

The astringent divining rod that relieves inflammation, bruises, sprains, and bleeding hemorrhoids

The *witch* part of the witch hazel (*Hamamelis virginica*) refers to the use of its branches as divining rods to locate underground water and ore. Liniment made from witch hazel inner bark and twigs soothes bruises, sprains, and other painful spots. Liniment made from the leaves stimulates the peripheral blood flow around parts of the body near the surface, thus lessening inflammation and relieving water-swollen tissues. American Indians made poultices of the inner bark to soothe their painfully inflamed eyes. Witch hazel's astringent leaves control diarrhea and, applied as a lotion, ease bleeding hemorrhoids. The tannins, ethereal oil, and probably also a saponin, account for witch hazel's anti-inflammatory and astringent properties.

Tea is brewed in the usual way, that is, pour 1 cup of boiling water over 1 teaspoonful of leaves or bark and steep 5 minutes before straining.

Medicine chest of 29 plants for alleviating wounds, infections, burns, and other skin conditions

Plant	Use
Aloe	Leaf juice relieves X-ray burns, sunburn, eczema, dermatitis, conjunctivitis and inflamed eyelids, skin ulcers
Arnica	Tincture (prepared according to instructions elsewhere in this book) on sprains and open wounds
Ash and perhaps other species)	Mucilage-rich bast fibers or inner bark strips help heal wounds when applied
Birch	Young crushed leaves applied to wounds and insect bites and stings
Burdock	Root decoction to stimulate hair growth
Camomile	Flower tea (1 to 2 tablespoonsful in a pint of water) for boils, inflammation
Candleberry or wax myrtle	Whole plant decoction applied to control bleeding
Carrot	Grated fresh carrot applied to burns, sores and frostbitten spots. Some people boil carrot until soft for packing on fetid sores.

Comfrey or bruisewort	Root decoction, root and/or leaf powder, or root and/leaf poultice for wounds, bruises, old sores. Root powder controls bleeding of fresh wounds. Comfrey favorably affects the periosteum (membrane that covers bone), hence its other name—knitbone.
Coneflower (narrow-leaved purple coneflower)	Root decoction applied to abscesses and boils
Daisy	Crushed flower applied to wounds and chapped skin
Elder	1 teaspoonful of leaves boiled in 1 cupful of water about 3 minutes and applied as wet dressing to burns
Flax	Flax or linseed oil mixed with lime water (that is, calcium hydroxide) and applied to relieve burn pain. Lime (also called burnt lime, calx or quicklime) is calcium oxide before water turns it into calcium hydroxide. Use only a medical grade; ask your pharmacist. Salt and flaxeed poultice for foul sores
Fumitory	Foliage tea applied to chronic eczema and to inflamed eye
Gentian	Root decoction as wet dressing on poorly healing or purulent wounds
Horsetail	Foliage tea applied to eczema, ulcers, sores, bone caries
Linden	Powdered charcoal from wood sprinkled on sores and purulent skin conditions
Lungwort	Decoction of powdered root and lower leaves, or the dry powder, applied to wound edges and inflammations
Madder	Root decoction (1 to 2 grams in cupful of water) or cold extract (by soaking a few grams overnight in cold water) or prepared as the Italian artist's friends did it for their urinary stones in Section 2, and applied to skin sores
Marigold	Flower tea applied to sebaceous cysts and inflamed sores, purulent gaping wounds, and wounds in which arnica would inflame and blister (which overly strong arnica tincture could do)

Melilot or yellow sweet clover	Flowering foliage tea (1 pint of boiling water poured over 1 tablespoonful) to soften and combat pain and inflammation in sores and boils
Mullein	Leaves and flowers as tea applied to soften and reduce pain in sores, wounds and external hemorrhoids
Onion	Boiled or roasted onion applied to soften and mature sores
Pansy	Foliage tea (1 tablespoonful boiled 3 minutes in cupful of water and steeped 10 minutes before application to eczema)
Plantain	Crushed leaves applied to fresh wounds and scrapes for relief
Ribgrass or lance-leaf plantain	Crushed leaves applied to bleeding wounds, scrapes, poorly healing old wounds, eczema
Saint John's wort	Although this plant can photosensitize some people, thus causing their skin to burn in the sun (temporarily), the plant's red oil has been used to apply to burns, sores and other skin conditions for relief.
Stinging nettle	Foliage tea applied to nervous eczema and other skin eruptions. Root boiled in vinegar applied to encourage hair growth and combat dandruff
Turnip	Poultice of ground-up turnip seeds applied nightly to lighten and/or clear up moles

A Bahamian herbalist's medicine chest

A Miami anthropologist/epidemiologist and a fourth generation herbalist from the Bahama Islands, just eastward of Miami, provided me with information from which I selected some of the plants most likely to be growing or at least known in the U.S. This should be read for interest only, and not used as a guide to self-medication unless under the supervision of a physician with herbal knowledge.

English name	Scientific name	How used
Aloe	*Aloe vera*	Jelly-like leaf pulp applied to

		soothe rashes, boils, minor wounds, insect stings and bites, acne and facial blemishes. Eaten with salt for respiratory conditions (colds, tuberculosis, etc.) and to stimulate appetite.
Bay geranium	*Ambrosia hispida*	White leaves boiled to make tea, drunk for colds, indigestion, weaknesses, and to retard aging. Tea mixed with lime and salt is drunk as tonic and to relieve pain. Tea applied as wet dressing on skin irritations.
Bay hop	*Ipomoea pescaprae*	Crushed leaves boiled for tea to relieve tiredness. Tea is added to bath water to alleviate sores and various wounds.
Bay rum	*Pimenta racemosa*	Leaves soaked in boiling water and resulting tea poured into bath water for skin cooling bath. For a stimulant, leaf tea is drunk, or dried leaves are rubbed on the forehead, or dried and powdered leaves are inhaled like snuff. Toasted (or parched) leaves are rubbed right on minor skin irritations.
Cascarilla	*Croton eluteria*	Leaves and bark boiled to make a tea drunk to sharpen senses and build resistance to disease.
Cerasee	*Momordica charantia*	Tea boiled from leaves and vine drunk hot with lemon and salt before breakfast to relieve colds, fever or diabetes (in which case it reportedly reduces the amount of sugar in the blood).

Goat pepper	*Capsicum frutescens*	Reddish fruit (the peppers) eaten to improve mental and physical powers, and to clear up congested throat.
Life leaf	*Bryophyllum pinnatum*	Leaf tea drunk to alleviate asthmatic shortness of breath (but also shortness of breath associated with other respiratory conditions), kidney conditions, boils and other skin infections (on which the tea is used as a wet dressing).
Lignum vitae	*Guaiacum officinale*	Leaf tea drunk regularly to cleanse and strengthen body, as antidote for poisoning (a use no doubt related to the cathartic effect of the bark and laxative effect of the blue flowers). Baths containing white sap from the bark added to bath to relieve pain.
Lime	*Citrus aurantifolia*	Fresh juice gargled for sore throat. Tea boiled from leaves drunk to reduce high blood pressure.
Mexican poppy	*Argemone mexicana*	Sap from snapped off stem rubbed on ringworm (which is really a fungus, not a worm) and on warts to remove them. Thick tea boiled down from whole plant (including roots) is drunk for hepatitis and to normalize urine flow. To prevent overdosage, avoid use unless under the guidance of a physician with herbal knowledge; the anthropologist who told me about this, said none of the Bahamians he knew about who used these remedies (as prepared and pre-

		scribed by the local herbalist) had any unpleasant reactions from them.
Papaya	*Carica papaya*	Fruit eaten to relieve constipation, and the glistening black seeds chewed for easing digestion. Also used to tenderize meat (see section on papaya earlier in this book).
Pencil tree	*Euphorbia tirucalli*	Sap from cut branches left on warts for "some time" then scrubbed off with the warts.
Pigeon plum	*Coccoloba diversifolia*	The plant's black berries are eaten to control diarrhea and increase stamina. Bark decoction drunk to alleviate pain. A Miami attorney, who suffered the miseries of ciguatera poisoning from a grouper he caught for dinner in the Gulfstream, told me he relieved his nausea, tingling fingers and lips, dizziness, disrupted vision and malaise overnight by drinking a cupful or so of a decoction of pigeon plum root mixed with a shot of gin.
Prickly pear	*Opuntia stricta*	Shampoo with crushed plant to clear up dandruff. Boiled leaves eaten to calm digestive upsets. Slices of the purplish fruit applied to painful arthritic and rheumatic spots.
Spanish "lime" or guinep	*Melicocca bifuga*	Fruit eaten to regulate blood pressure and to spark appetite.

Much of the information in the above table was kindly made available by Dr. Robert Halberstein, Chairman of the Department of Anthropology, University of Miami, Coral Gables, Florida.

Section 3

Introduction to Blended Plant Recipes for Enhanced Healing Powers

Combination remedies or "recipes" are good because the plants in them can reinforce, tone down, release, trigger, or otherwise alter the effects of each other in the mixture. A mixture of several plants can offer more healing or protective powers than any one of the separate plants in the mixture could do alone—that is, *the whole is greater than the sum of its parts*, just as it is with a human being, who is much more than brain + heart + liver and so on. A Swiss scientist, Emil Bürgl, gave us the rule that two or more medications with the same effect, but with different points of action in the body, *potentiate* each other when used together, that is, their combined effect is more powerful than the sum of the powers from each plant in the combination. Every good cook and baker who combines tasteless or inedible items to prepare delicious and nutritious meals understands the value of combining and blending ingredients for best results.

A disagreeable or overly strong plant is often mixed with other plants that improve its flavor or make it safer to take. Another advantage of combinations is that they can be used over longer periods without alternating with other remedies or teas, as is advisable with single-plant teas and remedies; use over long periods of some teas with only one plant in them, or without switching over now and then to another plant, could lead to irritation or other inconveniences.

Two plant recipes thousands of Europeans use for biliary and digestive health

The following plant recipes are examples of combinations which proved successful for two reasons: the plants in them mutually reinforce and/or control each other, and their "shotgun" approach stands a better chance of hitting an uncertain target. That is, if you know it's your liver or gallbladder, but don't know whether its more the one or the other, or if you suspect it's just that greasy, fat-heavy banquet that messed up your digestion, then combination recipes may help. In any case, these kinds of combinations have been used successfully at home and in the hospital on patients with biliary conditions. If you suspect a serious condition or have a frightening emergency, however, then for heaven's sake do *not* rush to learn everything about herbal medicine all at once, but get a physician's help or at least advice—you can always disagree with his or her treatment later, or even suggest that he or she try the herbal remedy out on your case. Many good physicians the world over recognize the possible merits of plant medicine. If the doctor smirks or shakes his or her head when you say you're going to mix up the remedy yourself, then you can always fall back on one of the professionally (that is, safely, conveniently and economically) compounded natural herbal remedies available on the market.

The twelve plants in the first combination remedy are (1) artichoke, (2) buckbean, (3) calamus, (4) camomile, (5) dandelion, (6) fennel, (7) gentian, (8) goldenseal, (9) holy thistle, (10) milfoil, (11) Saint Benedict's thistle, and (12) wormwood, plus fructose or fruit sugars. Why did pharmacologists and herb-wise physicians choose these twelve plants and fructose? Here are the reasons:

Artichoke promotes liver function by stimulating the secretion of bile and promoting its natural flow through the biliary system, and in this way fosters healthy digestion of fats and prevents gallstones. *Dandelion* and *holy thistle* reinforce these effects of artichoke. (Holy thistle also supports the liver's detoxifying powers. Dandelion is also great for maintaining a healthy urinary flow.)

Buckbean contributes by fostering the flow of digestive juices, just as *calamus* does. Calamus, in addition, guards against other distressful things such as overacidity, gas, diarrhea, and cramps. The relief of cramps, however, is camomile's specialty, but it also fights inflammation and gas. *Fennel* is another cramp and gas reliever from way back in history.

Besides buckbean, the other bitters in this combination are *gentian, Saint Benedict's thistle* and *wormwood,* all of which work wonders with digestion.

Milfoil, like camomile, is an effective all-round helper that aids digestion, reduces inflammation and cramping, and gets rid of gas.

The natural *fruit sugar* or *fructose* which takes the edge off some of the bitter taste in this recipe, is a natural sweetner of which even diabetics have little to fear. Fructose is made into bread for diabetics, as a matter of fact, because this natural sugar is readily metabolized in the body, with no undue stress on the liver, into glycogen (often called animal starch) even when insulin is lacking. So, besides pleasantly sweetening up some of the bitterness of the other plants in this combination, fruit sugars also protect the liver and the organs that work with it.

If you want to make this remedy yourself instead of purchasing it ready-made, then measure out (or have a druggist do it for you) the following amounts of well dried and stored plant parts:

Artichoke leaves	3.0 grams
Buckbean leaves	0.07 gram
Calamus rootstock	0.15 gram
Camomile flowers	0.4 gram
Dandelion foliage	1.0 gram
Fennel "seed" (really fruit)	0.4 gram
Fruit sugars or fructose	18.0 grams
Goldenseal rhizome (Don't collect yourself; don't use more than specified. (See note page 135.)	0.6 gram
Gentian root	0.8 gram
Holy thistle "seeds" (really fruit	0.4 gram
Milfoil foliage	0.6 gram
Saint Benedict's thistle foliage	0.15 gram
Wormwood foliage	0.04 gram

The German apothecary who told me about this one recommended this way of preparing a tea from the above mix: bring 100 milliliters (or about 3 ounces) of water containing the harder ingredients (rootstock, rhizome and crushed "seeds") to a boil in an enameled pot or in a pyrex glass pot. (The idea is not to have any bare metal contact the plants.) Add a little more water to bring the whole amount back up to about 3 or 4 ounces. Bring quickly to a boil again and pour (while still boiling) over the other ingredients (leaves, flowers, foliage). Cover and let steep about 10 minutes. Take 1 or 2 tablespoonsful with or just after each meal. (This remedy is not recommended if you suffer from severe liver disorders, biliary obstruction, purulent gallbladder inflammation, or severe liver insufficiency.)

What's in another popular German plant remedy for liver, gallbladder and digestive health? In addition to the artichoke, camomile, holy thistle and dandelion mentioned, there's boldo, peppermint, narrow-leaved purple coneflower, rose hips, wheat germ, papain, rhubarb, yeast, valerian, tumeric, and lecithin.

Boldo, tumeric and *peppermint* reinforce the effects of artichoke. (Boldo also supports the liver's role of neutralizing and/or eliminating toxins. Peppermint also eases digestive distress, and tumeric relaxes cramps in the gallbladder's sphincter of Oddi.)

The *narrow-leaved purple coneflower* bolsters the body's natural resistance, thus aids the liver in its defense of the body against environmental poisons. *Yeast*, too, supports the body's natural resistance to disease, as well as provides a load of vitamins, enzymes, and other vital substances.

Wheat germ is a concentrated shot of vitamin E (anti-sterility and anti-muscular dystrophy vitamin), vitamin F (essentially fatty acids), and other substances.

Rose hips contribute a great deal of vitamin C as well as a general beneficial effect on the gallbladder.

Papain, the enzyme from *papaya*, promotes digestion, especially of proteins, and works along with peppermint and camomile to keep the digestive processes running smoothly all the way to the small intestine.

Rhubarb takes care of maintaining healthy intestinal activity—guarding against diarrhea as well as constipation.

Valerian sedates an overly excitable nervous system, thereby calms down colicky pains and cramping, and helps provide a good night's sleep.

The natural cholin from *soybean* lecithin, a known liver protector, promotes and activates healthy function of liver cells and bolsters the liver's work of detoxifying all the poisons that pass through us every day.

To prepare this combination yourself, you'd need some experience in brewing and extracting from plant materials, and some way to measure out and make into tablets or pills the substances you extract from the plants. So, I think the best thing to do with this one is to make a tea mixture from the same kinds of plants in the tablets, and drink a few sips of it after meals. Here's what goes into the remedy:

Artichoke leaves	40 pinches
Boldo leaves	12 pinches
Camomile flowers	24 pinches
Narrow-leaved purple coneflower	24 pinches
Dandelion foliage	24 pinches
Holy thistle "seed"	24 pinches
Papain (buy this extract ready-made)	10 pinches
Peppermint leaves	12 pinches
Rhubarb root	12 pinches
Rose hips	20 pinches
Soy lecithin (buy this extract ready-made)	10 pinches
Tumeric rhizome	48 pinches
Valerian root	10 pinches
Wheat germ (buy this extract ready-made)	30 pinches
Yeast (buy fresh)	30 pinches

Note: This remedy is not recommended if you suffer from severe liver disorders, biliary obstruction, purulent gallbladder inflammation, or severe liver insufficiency.

Vein teas, tablets, and baths that help heal vein problems

Teas and other herbal remedies are often prescribed by physicians in many parts of the world as supplemental treatment along with other therapy. A clinical test in Germany, for example, showed the effect on 36 women and 24 men of a herbal tea plus herbal tablets plus herbal baths available in Europe for improving venous perfusion and firming up vessel walls, and, in general helping clear up vein problems (such as varicose veins, venous stagnation, and leg ulcers).

Each patient received a nine-week course of treatment with tea, tablets, and baths: 2 tablets 3 times a day, 1 cup of tea 3 times a day, and 2 baths a week. After nine weeks the physician observed improvements in his patients movements, calf circumference, size and condition of their leg ulcers, blood sedimentation rate, and numbers of white blood cells.

The vein tablets contained extracts of gingko leaves, Chinese yellow berry buds, horse chestnuts, witch hazel leaves, milfoil, rhubarb, rose hips, Indian valerian, arnica flowers and vitamin B1. The vein baths contained extracts of milfoil, oak bark, horse chestnut and camomile flowers, as well as wheat germ oil, Siberian pine oil, carotene-containing vegetable oil, soybean lecithin, yeast tincture, chlorophyll, and a coconut oil foamer.

Vein tablets and medicinal bath extracts can be obtained from health food stores and distributors. So can tea mixtures. But tea mixes can also be put together at home, too. The tea used in the medical test described above contains the following plants:

16 grams horse chestnut leaves
 7 grams marigolds
 8 grams night-blooming cereus flowers
 5 grams stinging nettle foliage
 5 grams with hazel leaves
 9 grams elder flowers
 8 grams pansies
 9 grams rose hips

9 grams sunflowers
9 grams milfoil flowers
8 grams strawberry leaves
7 grams lemongrass

One reputable international firm which mixes herbal remedies recommends pouring 1 cup of boiling water over 1 heaping table-spoonful of the above mixture and drinking 2 or 3 cups a day.

A six-essential oil "cure all" mixture used by Chinese, Europeans, and Americans

Here are over a dozen personal experiences of physicians, dentists and their patients who used Basle oil (oleum basileum or Olbas, a European version of the centuries-old Chinese po-ho remedy)—a mixture of the essential oils of peppermint, eucalyptus, melaleuca (cajeput or bottle-brush tree), juniper, clove, and wintergreen. Note that this oil is named after *Basle*, a Swiss city, and not the spice herb *basil*.

Drunkenness. A drinker's friend reports: "Although I can't explain it, the fact remains that a few drops of Basle oil taken with water can clear up a severely drunk person's mind and restore his bodily balance, at least temporarily so you can help get him home more or less under his own power. Even in the worse cases, I was always able to count on about a 15- to 20-minute grace period of calmness and tractibility in my friend's drunkeness during which time we managed to get him home safely."

Laryngitis. Mr. D.'s dry, irritated throat was indeed a "pain in the neck" because for months it had been keeping him from properly controlling his classroom of vociferous high school students. The more he tried to speak, the more they laughed at his piping, cracking voice. Even the school doctor ran out of ways of trying to soothe Mr. D.'s throat and restore his voice. Finally, the school custodian, who had emigrated from Switzerland years before, handed the perplexed teacher a bottle containing a mixture of six essential or ethereal oils—Basle oil. The teacher rubbed a few drops of it into his neck and inhaled some of it (2 drops of the pure oil, not the paraffin-based ointment form, in a pan of boiling water), afterwards wiping his face dry and keeping it warm. He felt some relief, but he still didn't have his voice back yet. He repeated this treatment the next day, and also repeated it again the day after that. After these three days, however, he was his own self again; his laryngitis was completely gone.

Note about pneumonia caused by inhalation of paraffin-based ointments: So-called lipoid pneumonia has been caused by inhalation of vapors from ointments or salves containing lipoids (fats or oils, including petrolatum products). A chunk of such lipoid-containing ointment dropped into boiling water vaporizes into microscopically tiny droplets. In fact, any form of heat at the boiling point, such as in the frying pan in your kitchen, sends fat droplets flying. That's how we get a greasy film on kitchen walls and ceiling. The vaporized lipoid droplets are so tiny that the sweeper cells (special cells with little whip-like filaments) along the respiratory tract can't brush them out, and the lungs can't handle them either, thus leading to pneumonia. It's the great heat which makes the oil-containing substances unsuitable for inhalation from boiling water, but they are quite safe when our own body heat evaporates them, such as when applied to the inside of the nose.

Burning tongue. A doctor reports: "For his burning, inflamed tongue, I had my patient rinse his mouth with ten drops of Basle oil in a glass of warm water until the pain subsided. Then I painted his tongue with undiluted oil. The benefit was almost immediate, and my method led to a surprisingly complete cure."

Tooth and gum abscess. A dental surgeon reports: "Soon after a 15-year-old girl had her upper left incisor filled, the filling began to irritate the pulp down in the tooth, and it became inflamed and infected. When I arrived (in those days I made house calls like any conscientious doctor or dentist, and I kept right on making them until I was 82), the poor girl was in bed, running a fever, her whole face swollen and painfully sensitive to the touch. The incisor was literally imbedded in a cushion of pus. I painted the surrounding gum with Basle oil, gently massaged some into the skin over the affected side of her face, and gave her a few drops to take in a tablespoon of warm water. The pain stopped. I left my patient with instructions for her parents to repeat the treatment. About three hours later, the pus burst out of the gum next to the tooth. Later, when she came to my office, I was able to save her tooth with a root canal procedure."

Pyorrhea (inflamed and infected gums). A dentist reports: "My patient's gums were badly inflamed, and after a week of painfully waiting for it to go away, pus began to form. He massaged Basle oil into the painful spots. Two days later, in preparation for his visit to my dental clinic at the university to see if he still had any infection, he told me he was able to brush his teeth vigorously without any pain at all. When I saw his gums, I was happy to tell him that his oil apparently had actually healed the inflamed pus-laden gums, and not just stopped his immediate pain."

Note on the use of medicines through the skin: Rubbing a remedy on the temples or behind the ears is not merely as "psychological" as it may seem to some skeptics. Even highly sophisticated drug firms are now developing and selling transdermal (through-the-skin) forms of medicine for applying to the patient's skin, from where the active ingredients enter into the body's various systems. So rubbing a remedy into the skin is certainly not an obsolete practice to be thrown out with some of granny's other health ideas. (In fact, the careful observer will see more and more of those "old-fashioned" techniques showing up in modern medicine. There is indeed not very much new under the sun.)

Sinusitis. A surgeon-shy doctor reports: "I was able to clear up purulent sinusitis in sixteen patients by rubbing Basle oil into the skin over the sinus areas four or five times spread out over two days' time, putting a few drops into the ears, applying warm compresses (sprinkled with twenty-five drops of the oil) over the sinus areas, and giving the patients a few drops of the oil on a lump of sugar. My treatment was always successful by the eighteenth to twentieth day. This success saved my patients from any surgery."

Asthma. An asthma sufferer reports: "For years I've been making the doctor rounds for my asthma. One day, a 95-year-old Swiss-Italian doctor (who painted landscapes in Wisconsin instead of practicing medicine) gave me a flask of Basle oil. I rubbed ten drops of it into my chest, and that night I covered up my chest with a warm, moist flannel cloth on which I first sprinkled fifteen to twenty drops of the oil. I broke out in the wettest sweat I've ever had. Finally, I breathed easier after three days of this day-night procedure. Then, I did it only once a week. In six weeks I felt and worked as if I had never suffered from asthma.

"That landscape-painting doctor told me two other ways he had used the oil successfully himself for alleviating the asthma of others:

1. In sixteen minutes his patient was breathing easier after he rubbed the oil over the heart and into the groove along the collar bone.

2. The patient took eight drops of the oil in a tablespoon of water twice a day. Then she massaged ten drops of it into her chest, throat and forehead. That same night she sprinkled seventeen drops of the oil on a warm, moist linen cloth and placed it around her chest. She breathed easily that night for the first time in a long while."

Hair loss and growth. A physician reports: "For years one of my patients had a large balding spot on the very top of his head. He was always showing me all the hair-growing remedies he was forever trying out, and I was always reminding him of their uselessness (not to speak of his vanity in hiding his baldness). Yet, a new experience was in store for me, his old doctor. A few weeks after he began rubbing Basle oil into his scalp, I saw new hair in his previously bald spot · Perhaps his baldness was due to some condition that was helped by the oil, I don't know. But I did see new hair growing out from his scalp."

Bladder stones. A doctor reports: "My patient was 65 years old and suffered from bladder stones. Our experiment with Basle oil was as follows: every day for eight days she took a hot bath (half bath or sitz bath) containing ten to twenty drops of Basle oil. Morning and evening she took five drops of the oil in a tablespoon of warm water. This led to a powerful urge to urinate (the urine giving her the impression that it was very warm) and an abundant flow of sand-like matter in her urine. Twelve days later my patient had colicky pains, for which we at once laid hot packs sprinkled with Basle oil over her abdomen, bladder and back. The pains subsided, but her urge to urinate grew steadily stronger. Two hours later, two grape-sized stones washed out in the stream of urine."

Quivering amputation stump. An amputee reports: "Four years ago my right leg was amputated because of tuberculosis in it. The stump healed but remained somewhat swollen, and the nerves made it quiver and jerk when the weather changed. I massaged the stump twice a day with Basle oil then wrapped it airtight with flannel or linen for awhile to build up some warmth. In a week or so the quivering and jerking stopped and didn't happen anymore for minor weather changes, unless a particularly violent change in weather came along, at which time I simply repeated the oil treatment for relief."

Leg cramps. After too vigorous a day of golf, Dr. L. massaged Basle oil into his leg (calf) muscles to relieve cramping. Relief was obtained almost at once.

Rheumatic back. Mrs. H.G. suffered so badly from rheumatism in her back, especially in the small of her back, that she found it difficult to walk or do almost anything at all. Eight days after she began rubbing the six-oil mixture into her back, her pain cleared up. This relief lasted at least thirty days (that was when she called her doctor to cancel her scheduled rheumatism treatment because she was too busy doing all her household chores).

Arthritis. A woman who had been hobbling along on an arthritically painful ankle massaged Basle oil into her ankle, then wrapped it loosely in flannel. Also, she took one or two drops of the oil on a lump of sugar. A few weeks and a few treatments later, her ankle joint was painless, allowing her to walk comfortably without hobbling.

Shaking hand. Mr. B. was a civil servant whose right hand weakened and began to tremble so severely that he was unable to write. Frequent massage with Basle oil for several days left his hand well enough to write as much as he needed to write during a full day at the office.

Phlebitis (inflamed veins) and varicose veins. Mrs. S. suffered from chronic phlebitis and varicose veins so painful that she could hardly move about the house. A few days after she massaged Basle oil into her legs, the pain and inflammation subsided. By the eighth day all swelling and pain were gone, and she had no difficulty in walking around as much as she desired.

Preliminary Note to Sections 4 Through 12

The remedies on the following pages were collected from (1) physicians who were familiar with the uses and effects of the plants in healthy and ill people, from (2) pharmacists who have compounded herbal remedies and who are therefore familiar with the official uses of the plants in their respective countries, and from (3) laboratories which produce remedies approved by the health authorities of their respective countries, many of which permit the scientifically valid medical and health uses of the plants to be clearly stated by the manufacturer, who is merely transmitting the traditional knowledge of the known effects of those plants.

Most of these teas, rinses, baths, and other combinations can be mixed up in your kitchen once you have the right parts of the right plants in the right condition and strength.

If you don't collect the plant fresh, then you can purchase it dried and cleanly packaged at local health food stores, and fresh from your local grocery and farmer. The main problem, however, is that the full curative and/or health powers of many plants come only from naturally grown plants. So, unless you grow your own, or know who grows what you use, you have to do the best with what's available. There are herbal pharmaceutical companies that produce and sell the combinations ready-made as dry teas in various forms, tablets and capsules, elixirs, tinctures, wines, medicinal baths, and extracts. If your local shops don't carry what you want, see the list in the appendix of this book for names and addresses of distributors and manufacturers of herbal remedies.

Note: The recipes in these sections include a few plants which should be used only in those recipes, professionally prepared in safe amounts and in the proper forms by reputable laboratories such as those listed in the appendix of this book. You may even want to

discuss it with your doctor. Such plants are arnica (see note under
the arnica table page 27), peony, toothpick plant, bittersweet
nightshade, tansy, juniper, larkspur (at least avoid seeds and young
plants), goldenseal, violetroot, European mistletoe, celandine.

Note: The best rule for safe recipes that act as effectively as
possible, is to obtain them pre-mixed from the reputable
laboratories and firms listed in the appendix. If a pre-mixed recipe is
available from these sources, then you'll find the name of the
formula (such as Dr. Greither formula, Galama formula, etc.) with
the recipe. Then find that name in the list of laboratories and firms.

Most of the plants in the recipes have already been mentioned
earlier with their scientific names (which you should use to avoid
confusion when dealing with unfamiliar plants). In any case, the
scientific names of all the plants are given in the index.

Section 4

Mouthwashes, Gargles, Rinses, Wet Compresses, Teas, Plasters, Rubs, Syrups, and Inhalations to Alleviate Mouth, Throat, and Chest Problems

Mouthwash for sore mouth

Soak one teaspoonful of the following mixture in one cup of cold water for about three hours, then bring the water and its contents to a boil. Strain and rinse the mouth with it:

1 teaspoon fennel seed
3 teaspoons oak bark
3 teaspoons sage leaves
3 teaspoons tormentil root

Six general gargles and mouthwashes

1. Garble with a tea made from a teaspoonful of the following mixture:

1 part elder flowers
1 part mallow flowers
1 part marshmallow leaves

2. Gargle hourly with a tea made from a teaspoonful of the following mixture:

1 part elder flowers
1 part mallow flowers
1 part sage leaves

3. Gargle hourly with a lukewarm tea made from two teaspoonsful of the following mixture:
1 part mallow leaves
1 part sage leaves
1 part tormentil root

4. Gargle with a tea made from a teaspoonful of the following mixture:
1 part oak bark
1 part sage leaves
1 part tormentil root

5. Gargle with a tea from one teaspoonful of the following mixture:
1 part blackberry leaves
1 part coltsfoot leaves
1 part mallow leaves
1 part sage leaves

6. Gargle with a tea from a teaspoonful of the following mixture:
5 teaspoons camomile flowers
1 teaspoon fennel seed
5 teaspoons peppermint leaves
5 teaspoons sage leaves

Inhalation for upper respiratory infections

Breathe in the vapors several times a day of a boiling pot (fireproof glass, enameled, stainless steel, or coated pots) of the following mixture in several cups of water:
2½ ounces camomile flowers
1 ounce thyme foliage

Be careful not to burn yourself with the *live* steam—that's the invisible part of the heat between the spout of the kettle and the visible cloud of condensed steam which you inhale.

Pharyngitis tea

Brew a tea from two teaspoonsful of a mixture of equal parts of aniseed and coltsfoot leaves. You can add a bit more coltsfoot leaves if you care to make the tea more soothing and less antiseptic. That's one of the advantages of mixing up herbal remedies once you become familiar with plants and their effects. Sweeten with honey and drink one cup hot every hour or so.

Another pharyngitis tea can be brewed from goldenrod foliage and drunk 3 times a day.

Laryngitis tea

Brew a tea from balm of Gilead buds (*Populus gileadensis*) 3 times a day.

Tea for sore throats, coughs and colds

Brew tea from elder flowers and drink about 4 cups a day as hot as you can.

Wet compresses for jaw abscesses

Brew a tea from the following mixture in a quart of water, and apply warm to the abscess:

> 1 ounce balm or melissa leaves
> 1 ounce marjoran foliage
> 1 ounce oregano foliage
> 1 ounce peppermint leaves
> ¼ ounce camomile flowers
> ¼ ounce elder flowers
> ¼ ounce lavender flowers

If it's too hard to calculate ¼ ounce, then mix up 20 pinches each of the balm, marjoran, oregano, and peppermint, plus 5 pinches each of camomile, elder and lavender.

Tea for cough caused by pharyngitis or laryngitis

Brew a tea from a tablespoonful of the following mixture:

1 part aniseed
1 part fennel seed
2 parts mallow leaves

Bronchial cough

Elecampane root tea 3 times a day.

Cough, phlegm, cold

Three cups of linden flower tea. Add several teaspoonsful of honey to sweeten.

Dry cough

Hoarehound leaf and flower tea 3 times a day.

Phlegm, hoarseness and bronchitis

Brew a tea from a teaspoonful of the following mixture:
1 part licorice root
1 part marshmallow root
2 parts Iceland moss

Cough from bronchitis and tracheitis

Brew a tea from 2 teaspoonsful of the following mixture and steep at least 15 minutes before sweetening with honey and drinking warm several times a day:
1 part aniseed
1 part coltsfoot leaves
1 part marshmallow root
1 part mullein flowers

Cough

Brew a tea from a teaspoonful of the following mixture:
1 part fennel seed (Crush just before mixing to liberate the ethereal or volatile oils.)

1 part Iceland moss
1 part licorice root
2½ parts marshmallow root
1½ parts plantain foliage
3 parts thyme leaves

Plaintain leaf alone, too, makes a cough tea; make it 3 times a day, and sweeten with honey.

Chronic bronchitis

Brew a tea from a teaspoonful of the following mixture:
1 part coltsfoot leaves
1 part elecampane root
1 part Iceland moss
1 part lungwort

Because this mixture contains hard (root) plant parts, boil the teaspoonful of it 10 or 15 minutes. The pharmacist who told me about this remedy suggested 3 cups a day.

Father Kneipp's cough tea

Father Sebastian Kneipp was a nineteenth century German priest who developed a system of healthful therapy based upon water, exercise, and herbal substances. Brew a tea with 1 teaspoonful of the following Kneipp cough tea mix·
1 part mullein flowers
1 part fenugreek
2 parts fennel seed
2 parts juniper berries (See note page 73.)
2 parts plantain leaves
2 parts mallow flowers
2 parts linden flowers
4 parts horsetail foliage
4 parts stinging nettle foliage
8 parts coltsfoot foliage

Chest plaster for croup

Cook 2 or 3 cloves of fresh garlic in 1 ounce of lard for half an hour at moderate heat. Apply warm to the chest and cover with a strip of clean muslin or other cloth. Remove in about an hour. If it seems to help, then repeat several hours later.

Throat and chest rub for cough

Massage the following mixture of oils into the throat and chest:
    2 drops eucalyptus oil
    2 drops rosemary oil
    2 drops thyme oil
    44 drops camphorated oil

Syrup for chronic cough

Boil handful of plantain (root, leaves, flowers or seeds) plus juniper berries* or fresh twigs in at least 1 quart of water for 3 hours. Strain out plant parts, add sugar, and continue boiling for several hours until syrup forms. An Italian engineer who worked in the sewers of a large city drank several cups of this syrup before breakfast, and several cups during the day to ease his chronic cough.

Laxative chest tea

Brew a tea from 1 teaspoonful of the following mixture (the Wegscheider formula):
    1 part senna leaves
    1 part walnut leaves
    4 parts fennel seed (Crush just before adding to the mixture.)
    7½ parts licorice root
    15 parts marshmallow root
    21½ parts crushed linseed

Two Austrian chest teas

1. Brew a tea from 1 teaspoonful of the following mixture:

---

*See Note page 73.

  1 part mallow flowers
  3 parts licorice root
  5 parts marshmallow root
  11 parts marshmallow leaves

2. Brew a tea from 1 teaspoonful of the following mixture:
  1 part crushed aniseed
  2 parts mallow flowers
  2 parts marshmallow leaves
  2 parts mullein flowers
  2 parts coltsfoot leaves
  2 parts thyme leaves
  4 parts marshmallow root
  5 parts licorice root

Two German chest teas

1. Brew a tea from 1 teaspoonful of the following mixture:
  1 part fennel seed (Crush just before adding to the mix.)
  2 parts licorice root
  7 parts marshmallow root

2. Brew a tea from 1 teaspoonful of the following mixture:
  1 part blue or poison flag rhizome (violetroot)
      (See note page 135.)
  2 parts mullein flowers
  2 parts crushed aniseed
  3 parts licorice root
  4 parts coltsfoot leaves
  8 parts marshmallow root

A Norwegian chest tea

Brew a tea from 1 teaspoonful of the following mixture:
  2 parts crushed aniseed
  3 parts coltsfoot leaves
  3 parts elder flowers
  6 parts licorice root
  6 parts marshmallow root

A Danish chest tea

If we add speedwell and mullein to the Norweigian formula above, we get the Danish version; brew like the above with 1 teaspoonful of the following mixture:

    2   parts of crushed aniseed
    3   parts of coltsfoot leaves
    3   parts licorice root
    3   parts mullein flowers
    3   parts speedwell flowers
    4   parts elder flowers
    4½ parts marshmallow root

A Swedish chest tea

Brew a tea from 1 teaspoonful of the following mixture:

    1 part crushed star anise (See caution about bastard or
        Japanese star anise in the section on anise, pages 24-25.)
    3 parts licorice root
    4 parts elder flowers
    6 parts hyssop foliage
    6 parts marshmallow root

A Belgian chest tea

Brew a tea from 1 teaspoonful of the following mixture:

    1 part everlasting flowers
    1 part mallow flowers
    1 part marshmallow flowers
    1 part mullein flowers

Seven teas to sweat out colds and the "flu"

1. Brew a tea from 2 teaspoonsful of the following mixture:
    1 part linden flowers
    1 part elder flowers

2. Brew a tea from 1 teaspoonful of the following mixture; 1 to 3 cups are drunk:

1 part linden flowers
1 part elder flowers
1 part mullein flowers

3. Brew 2 or 3 teaspoonsful of the following mixture in 8 ounces of water (be sure to let the tea steep about 10 minutes after you pour he boiling water over the mixture)·
1 part linden flowers
1 part elder flowers
1 part camomile flowers

Don't sip, but drink right down while hot.

4. Brew a tea from a teaspoonful of the following mixture:
1 part camomile flowers
1 part elder flowers
1 part cornflower foliage

5. Brew a tea from 2 teaspoonsful of the following mixture, letting the tea steep 3 minutes:
1 part birch leaves
1 part elder flowers
1 part linden flowers

6. Brew a tea from 1 teaspoonful of the following mixture:
1 part licorice root
2½ parts linden flowers
3 parts rose hips
3½ parts elder flowers

7. Brew a tea from 1 teaspoonful of the following mixture:
1 part camomile flowers
1 part elder flowers
1 part linden flowers
1 part peppermint leaves

Cough tea

Brew 1 to 2 cups a day from 2 grams of the following mixture (*Salus formula*) per cup:

15 grams fennel seed
14 grams aniseed
10 grams licorice root
 8 grams malabar nut tree leaves
 8 grams orange blossoms
 8 grams eucalyptus leaves
 8 grams elder flowers
 7 grams violetroot (Not from violet but *Iris* species. See note page 135.)
 7 grams mallow flowers
 7 grams mullein flowers
 4 grams hoarhound foliage
 4 grams soapwort root

Quite a few of the remedies in this section are also prepared in forms other than teas (some of which come in tea bags, some as soluble powders, and some as liquid concentrates in tubes). The above cough tea, for example, also comes as an alcoholic tincture which can be taken as drops or can be vaporized and inhaled as an aerosol. I've stressed the teas, however, because they are the simplest to mix up at home from plant parts. If you'd like to experiment with making your own tinctures at home, see the instructions on page 26.

Inhalations can be prepared from steaming teas as well as from tinctures. Vapor baths—once standard health care for American Indians, and still is for Indians in Mexico and elsewhere in Latin America, many Asians, and Scandinavians—can be prepared from concentrated plant oils. The Atzinger Leukona sauna concentrate formula contains 0.75 milligrams (a milligram is a thousandth part of a gram) thyme oil, 1.5 gram menthol (from peppermint), 7.25 grams camphor, 8 grams Siberian pine oil and 42.5 grams eucalyptus oil. About 30 drops of this mix are added to a quart of boiling water which then gives off its vapors, preferably in a sauna or dry hot-air bath the Finns prepare by dashing cold water over hot rocks.

Tea for tracheitis and bronchitis

Brew 1 cup of tea from a teaspoonful or so of the following mixture (Stada Dapulmon formula); this is done 3 times a day:

1 part cornflower
1 part everlasting
3 parts melilot foliage
5 parts thyme foliage
5 parts fennel seed
5 parts peppermint leaves
10 parts lance-leaf plantain foliage
10 parts marshmallow root
10 parts mallow flower
10 parts licorice root
20 parts lungwort foliage
20 parts coltsfoot leaves

Tea to strengthen bronchi and lungs during the cold-catching season

Brew a tea by pouring 1 cupful of boiling water over 1 teaspoonful to 1 tablespoonful of the following mixture (*Kühne formula*) which is drunk as needed:

4.1 parts aniseed
8.1 parts marshmallow root
4.1 parts fennel seed
4.1 parts elder flowers
40.8 parts coltsfoot leaves
6.1 parts mullein flowers
4.1 parts linseed
4.1 parts linden flowers
4.1 parts milfoil foliage
8.1 parts plantain foliage
4.1 parts licorice root
4.1 parts thyme foliage
4.1 parts horsetail foliage

To simplify this formula, just drop the fractions (that is, make it 4 instead of 4.1, but 41 instead of 40.8 because .8 is more than half), then divide by a common denominator (2 goes into them all), so the parts become· 2, 4, 2, 2, 21, 3, 2, 2, 2, 4, 2, 2, 2.

Bronchial tea for respiratory catarrh

For a tea that loosens phlegm, disinfects and soothes irritation as well as the urge to cough, several cups of the following tea (Dr. Greither formula) are drunk instead of other drinks throughout the day (pour ½ a pint of boiling water over 1 tablespoonful of the following mixture):

4 grams aniseed
3 grams arnica flowers (See note page 135.)
4 grams dill seeds
7 grams fennel seeds
3 grams elder flowers
9 grams coltsfoot leaves
5 grams Iceland moss
4 grams camomile flowers
4 grams mullein flowers
4 grams dwarf or mountain pine
6 grams linden flowers
5 grams sage leaves
4 grams milfoil flowers
3 grams cowslip or primrose flowers
2 grams white dead nettle flowers
6 grams knotgrass foliage
7 grams juniper berries (See note page 135.)
2 grams water fennel seeds
6 grams thyme foliage

Chest and cough tea with spasm-relieving effects

For a tea that loosens phlegm, disinfects and reduces cramping associated with convulsive or spasmodic coughing, cups of the following tea (Dr. Greither formula) are drunk several times a day (pour ½ a pint of boiling water over 2 tablespoons of the following mixture and steep 10 minutes in a covered container):

5 grams aniseed
1 gram arnica flowers (See note page 27.)
5 grams stinging nettle foliage

6 grams eucalyptus leaves
8 grams fennel seed
4 grams crampweed foliage
8 grams coltsfoot leaves
3 grams coltsfoot flowers
3 grams Saint John s wort foliage
5 grams Iceland .moss
6 grams mountain pine sprouts
4 grams linseed
4 grams linden flowers
3 grams mallow flowers
5 grams wild thyme foliage
2 grams marigolds
2 grams cowslip or primrose flowers
8 grams thyme foliage
8 grams juniper berries (See note page 135.)
3 grams water fennel seeds
2 grams mullein flowers

Tea to prevent attacks of bronchial asthma,
to alleviate irritation and cramping, to disinfect,
and to strengthen the connective tissues

Brew a tea by pouring 1 cupful of boiling water over 1 tablespoonful of the following mixture (Dr. Greither formula) 1 cup is drunk warm morning, noon and evening, or sometimes more often if necessary:

2 grams arnica flowers (See note page 27.)
6 grams stinging nettle foliage
6 grams fennel seed
10 grams raspberry leaves
3 grams elder flowers
3 grams coltsfoot flowers
9 grams Iceland moss
3 grams coriander seed
3 grams mallow flowers
3 grams peonies (See note page 135.)
5 grams orange blossoms

2 grams marigolds

8 grams rosemary leaves

3 grams primroses

3 grams centaury foliage

6 grams thyme foliage

9 grams water fennel

3 grams mullein flowers

5 grams toothpick or ammi plant (from which khellin, a bronchial and coronary dilator, is obtained. See note page 135.)

5 grams horsetail foliage

3 grams Arenaria

Because the above remedy contains peonies, and both of the above contain toothpick or ammi plant fruit (from which khellin, a bronchial and coronary dilator, is obtained), the two remedies should be used only when medically approved and professionally made.

Section 5

Combination Teas to Alleviate Heart and Circulatory Ailments, Rheumatic Distress, and Joint Pains

Tea for palpitations, insomnia, and gastrointestinal distress (especially gas)

Put a teaspoonful of the following mixture in a cupful of cold water, bring it to a boil, and drink it warm as needed:

3 parts lemon balm or melissa leaves
3 parts valerian root
4 parts milfoil foliage

Sweat-producing tea for heart muscle and valvular disorders along with arthritis

Brew a tea from a teaspoonful of the mixture below, and sip a cup throughout the day. If you do this more than on 2 or 3 successive days, then stop for about 4 days before starting again.

2 parts pansy foliage
2 parts violet foliage
3 parts elder flowers
3 parts linden flowers

Tea for angina pectoris and high blood pressure

Pour boiling water over 2 teaspoonsful of the following mixture and steep it for about 8 hours:

1 part camomile flowers
1 part hawthorn flowers
1 part European mistletoe (See note page 84.)
1 part valerian root

The physician who told me about this remedy said his patients benefited from drinking a cup of it in the morning and a cup in the evening for at least 4 weeks at a time.

Anti-sclerotic tea

Pour 1 cupful of boiling water over 1 to 2 teaspoonsfuls of the following mixture, steep at least half an hour but preferably overnight, and strain out the plant parts. A German physician recommended 3 cups a day for about 2 months in order to calm cramping and spasms ,in the arteries (but check first with your doctor before long-term use.)

2 parts crushed caraway seed
2 parts rue foliage (The various effects of rue include
     stimulation of menstruation; rue is not recommended for
     expectant mothers.)
3 parts lemon balm or melissa leaves
3 parts valerian root
4 parts hawthorn flowers
6 parts European mistletoe foliage and stems (See note page
     84.)

Another tea (3 cups a day) for protection against arteriosclerosis and high blood pressure is made by pouring 1 cupful of boiling water over 1 or 2 teaspoonsful of the following mixture and steeping it overnight:

1 part crushed fresh garlic
1 part European mistletoe foliage (See note page 84.)
1 part hawthorn flowers

Anti-arteriosclerotic tea for clearing up
or lessening rush of blood to the head,
dizziness, fatigue, heart palpitations,
ringing in the ears

Brew as usual (a cup of boiling water over a tablespoonful of the mixture) a tea from the following mixture (Mauermann formula):
 5 parts hawthorn leaves
 2 parts rosemary leaves
 3 parts black locust flowers (flowers have been used in Europe to season food)
 1 part black elder flowers
 4 part hawthorn fruit
 2 parts juniper berries (See note page 73.)
 3 parts horsetail

Artery tea for preventing and alleviating
hardening of the arteries, maintaining
normal blood pressure, and encouraging good
blood flow through the coronary arteries

Pour 1 cup of boiling water over 1 tablespoonful of the following mixture (Dr. Greither formula) and steep 10 minutes (1 to 2 cups a day are drunk):
 3 grams arnica flowers (See note page 27.)
 3 grams basil foliage
 3 grams watercress foliage
 3 grams biting stonecrop or wall pepper
 7 grams lemon balm or melissa leaves
 9 grams European mistletoe foliage (See note page 84.)
 3 grams orange blossoms
 8 grams milfoil flowers
 6 grams senna pods
 13 grams hawthorn leaves and flowers
 5 grams ammi or toothpick plant (See note page 135.)
 11 grams horsetail foliage
 3 grams hawthorn berries

Don't use in cases of intestinal obstruction, and expectant mothers should be cautions.

Anti-arteriosclerotic tea

Brew a day's 2 cups of tea by pouring 2 cupfuls of boiling water over 2 tablespoonsful of the following mixture (Ikabo formula), leaving the plant parts in the container throughout the day as you pour off each cup of tea. Later on, 3 or 4 cups may be drunk a day, keeping the same basic proportion of 1 tablespoon of mixture to 1 cupful of boiling water.

  9 grams boldo leaves
  8 grams birch leaves
  4 grams peppermint leaves
  2 grams blackberry leaves
  2 grams strawberry leaves
  9 grams milfoil blossoms
 13 grams juniper berries (See note page 73.)
  7 grams aniseed
  5 grams rose hips
  5 grams hawthorn berries
  4 grams caraway seed
  4 grams horsetail foliage
  7 grams parsley seed
  4 grams European mistletoe leaves and/or stems (See note
   page 84.)
  7 grams heather flowers
  3 grams everlasting
  1 gram larkspur

Tea to prevent circulatory disorders resulting from hardening of the arteries

Brew a tea by pouring 1 cupful of boiling water over 1 table-spoonful of the following mixture (Dr. Greither formula). A morning and an evening cup are drunk over extended periods.

  2 grams arnica flowers (See note page 27.)
  7 grams watercress foliage
  4 grams damiana leaves
  5 grams melissa leaves
  9 grams European mistletoe foliage (See note page 84.)
  3 grams parsley seed
  3 grams senna leaves

4 grams senna pods
4 grams milfoil flowers
8 grams juniper berries (See note page 73.)
16 grams hawthorn leaves and flowers
6 grams hawthorn berries
6 grams horsetail foliage

Heart-calming tea to promote circulation in the coronary vessels and calm down nervousness

One cup of the following tea is drunk in the morning and one in the evening (pour ½ a pint of boiling water over 1 tablespoonful of the following (Dr. Greither formula) mixture:

2 grams arnica flowers (See note page 27.)
5 grams goldenrod foliage
3 grams motherwort foliage
7 grams cactus (night-blooming cereus) blossoms
10 grams European mistletoe leaves (See note page 84.)
7 grams melissa or lemon balm leaves
10 grams rosemary leaves
4 grams milfoil flowers
3 grams meadowsweet flowers
5 grams knotgrass foliage
13 grams hawthorn leaves and flowers
7 grams hawthorn berries

Tea to promote excretion of uric acid in people predisposed to rheumatism

Brew a tea by pouring 1 cupful of boiling water over 1 teaspoonful to 1 tablespoonful of the following mixture (Kühne formula) and steep 5 to 10 minutes:

19.8 parts blackberry leaves
5.1 parts strawberry leaves
4.5 parts seedless rose hips
4.1 parts raspberry leaves
0.5 parts cornflowers

4.7 parts linden flowers
2   parts peppermint leaves
1   part marigolds
1.6 parts woodruff foliage
3   parts alder buckthorn bark
0.3 part fennel seed
0·1 part elder flowers
0.2 part camomile flowers
1.2 part milfoil foliage
3.3 parts senna leaves
1.6 parts senna pods
5.2 parts juniper berries (See note page 73.)
15   parts bean skins
13.1 parts stinging nettle foliage
1.2 parts everlasting flowers
2.5 parts horsetail foliage
2.5 parts birch leaves
2.5 parts maté leaves
2.5 parts black currant leaves
2.5 parts couchgrass rootstock

Rheumatism tea to flush out uric acid

Brew a tea by pouring 1 cupful of boiling water over a heaping tablespoonful of the following mixture (Galama formula):
12 grams birch leaves
4 grams juniper berries (See note page 73.)
7 grams milfoil
8 grams senna leaves
5 grams senna pods
4 grams everlasting flowers
8 grams willow bark
10 grams restharrow root
8 grams alder buckthorn bark
9 grams rose hips
5 grams bitter orange peel
6 grams red sandalwood
3 grams stinging nettle foliage
5 grams guaiac wood

Tea to maintain normal metabolism and ward off rheumatism by promoting urinary flow, intestinal and liver function

Pour 1 cup of boiling water over 1 tablespoonful of the following mixture (Dr. Greither formula) and steep 5 to 10 minutes (2 or 3 cups a day are drunk for extended periods)

12 grams dandelion leaves
10 grams horsetail foliage
10 grams milfoil flowers
10 grams stinging nettle leaves
10 grams fennel seed
 7 grams birch leaves
 7 grams senna leaves
 8 grams senna pods
 5 grams barberries
 5 grams mountain ash or rowan berries
 5 grams juniper berries (See note page 73.)
 5 grams linden flowers
 3 grams arnica flowers (See note page 27.)
 3 grams marigolds

Don't use in cases of intestinal obstruction, and expectant mothers should be cautions.

Rheumatism tea for supplementary therapy

Brew a tea from 2 tablespoonsful of the following mixture (Stada formula) by pouring 1 pint of boiling water over it and then boiling for another 10 minutes before straining out the plant parts; 1 cup is drunk hot every 2 hours:

1 gram cornflowers
1 gram marigolds
1 gram peonies (If you mix this remedy up yourself at home instead of buying it ready-made, omit the peonies. Inexperienced collection or use of this plant, as well as of bitter nightshade mentioned below, is unsafe·)
5 grams bittersweet nightshade (See above note·)
2 grams juniper berries (See note page 73.)

5 grams alder buckthorn bark
8 grams elder flowers
10 grams meadowsweet foliage
10 grams stinging nettle foliage
17 grams willow bark
20 grams horsetail foliage
20 grams birch leaves

Section 6

50 Remedies That Overcome Gastrointestinal Distress or Obesity

Anti-cramp tea

Brew a tea from 1 teaspoonful of the following mixture:
1 part milfoil foliage
2 parts orange blossoms
3 parts valerian root

Tea for queasy stomach and twinge of nausea

The unfortunate choice of restaurant in one of the places I recently visited caused me a day of digestive distress, which is not usual for me because I can eat almost anything. But this time the heavy, greasy food was poorly cooked, and hard traveling had lowered my resistance. In the garden of the person I was visiting, however, I found half a dozen kitchen spice plants, three of which settled my stomach within an hour:
Lemon balm or melissa
Peppermint
Sage
I plucked 2 or 3 leaves of each, crushed them and poured a cup of boiling water over them. After they steeped 5 minutes in a covered cup (simply covered with the saucer), I added a teaspoonful of honey and drank the whole thing while it was still warm.

A Moroccan tea to relieve indigestion

A Moroccan chemistry professor overcame his indigestion

following overly sumptuous feasts by sipping mouthfuls of a tea
made as follows:
1. Softening caraway (seeds) and thyme (foliage) in water
2. Adding fresh lemon juice
3. Adding freshly prepared sandarac resin (from the *Callitris
   quadrivalvis* or sandarac tree, whose resin is used to make
   dental cement, incense, varnish, etc.)
4. heating the mixture to the boiling point and holding it there
   several seconds

then pouring it in a cup and taking large sips (or gulps) while still hot
(but don't burn yourself—this gentleman was used to gulping down
hot coffee and tea).

North African drink to assuage stomach pain

A shop-keeper in a bazaar put a pinch of crushed cumin seed in a
glass of orange blossom water (made by soaking or heating orange
blossoms in water, or by steam-distilling them); 1 cupful in the
morning and 1 cupful in the evening eased his vague (probably
indigestion or nerves, he said) stomach pains, usually in an hour.

Four Austrian, German and Swiss aromatic
teas for digestion and nervous stomach

1. Brew 1 teaspoonful of the following mixture for 1 cup of tea in
the evening:
    1 part lavender flowers
    2 parts marjoram foliage
    3 parts peppermint leaves
    4 parts sage leaves

2. Brew 1 or 2 teaspoons of the following mixture for 1 or 2 cups
of tea after meals or in the evening:
    1 part Java pepper or cubeb unripe fruit. (Java pepper
        sometimes is smoked in cigarettes to relieve asthma or
        hayfever-like symptoms.)
    1 part clove flower buds

2 parts lavender flowers
2 parts peppermint leaves
2 parts thyme foliage
2 parts wild or mountain thyme foliage

3. Brew a teaspoonful of the following mixture and drink a half or whole cupful of it after eating:
1 part angelica root
1 part calamus root
1 part clove flower buds
1 part ginger root
1 part lavender flowers
1 part sage leaves
1 part wild or mountain thyme
1½ parts marjoram foliage
1½ parts peppermint leaves

4. Brew 1 tablespoonful of the following mixture in a cupful of water, steep 10 minutes in a covered cup, strain, and drink unsweetened and warm half an hour before meals:
1   part everlasting flowers
2½ parts calamus root
2½ parts gentian root
2½ parts valerian root
5   parts aniseed
5   parts camomile flowers
5   parts caraway seed
5   parts centaury foliage
5   parts fennel seed
7½ parts peppermint leaves
10   parts milfoil foliage

Gastrointestinal tea to promote good digestion and discourage gas

In addition to eliminating and preventing gas, this tea's bitter principles encourage stomach and intestinal digestive juices, and its mucilage soothes irritation as well as lubricates the movement of intestinal contents. It's made by pouring 1 cup of boiling water over 1 tablespoonful of the following mixture (Dr. Greither formula), and is drunk before meals and over extended periods):

4 grams aniseed
2 grams arnica flowers (See note page 27.)
1 gram buckbean leaves
4 grams dill seed
4 grams marshmallow leaves
5 grams fennel seed
2 grams psyllium seed
5 grams camomile flowers
4 grams coriander seed
4 grams caraway
6 grams lavender flowers
8 grams linseed
6 grams linden leaves
3 grams mallow flowers
4 grams peppermint leaves
3 grams peony flowers (See note page 135.)
4 grams orange blossoms
2 grams marigolds
3 grams sage leaves
2 grams dead white nettle flowers
1 gram centaury foliage
7 grams knotgrass foliage
8 grams juniper berries (See note page 73.)
8 grams horsetail foliage

Three Belgian, Swiss and Austrian bitter teas for encouraging digestive juices

1. Brew a tea from 1 teaspoonful of the following mixture:
   1 part centaury foliage
   1 part Saint Benedict's thistle foliage
   1 part wormwood foliage

2. Brew a tea from 1 teaspoonful of the following mixture:

1 part buckbean leaves
1 part centaury foliage
1 part orange peel (bitter, Seville or sour orange, *Citrus aurantium*)
1 part Saint Benedict's thistle foliage
1 part wormwood foliage

3. Brew a tea from 1 teaspoonful of the following mixture:
   1 part cinnamon bark
   2 parts buckbean leaves
   2 parts calamus root or rhizome
   4 parts centaury foliage
   4 parts orange peel
   4 parts wormwood foliage

Six teas to prevent and relieve gas

1. Brew a tea from 1 teaspoonful of the following mixture (crush the "seeds"):
   1 part aniseed
   1 part caraway seeds
   1 part coriander seeds
   1 part fennel seeds

2. Brew a tea from 1 teaspoonful of the following mixture:
   1 part calamus root
   1 part camomile flowers
   1 part caraway seed (crushed)
   1 part peppermint leaves

3. Brew a tea from 1 teaspoonful of the following mixture:
   1 part caraway seeds (crushed)
   3 parts camomile flowers
   3 parts peppermint leaves
   3 parts valerian root

4. Brew a tea from 1 teaspoonful of the following mixture after the evening meal and before going to bed:
   1 part calamus root or rhizome

1 part cardamon seed
2 parts valerian root
3 parts camomile flowers
3 parts peppermint leaves

5. Brew a tea from 1 tablespoonful of the following mixture:
1   part valerian root
1½ parts calamus root or rhizome
2   parts peppermint tea
2½ parts camomile flowers
3   parts caraway seed (crushed)

6. Brew a tea from 1 teaspoonful of the following mixture:
1 part camomile flowers
1 part fennel seeds (crushed)
2 parts couchgrass or couch-quitch rhizome
2 parts licorice root
2 parts marshmallow root

Powder or tea for gas, diarrhea, nausea, and vomiting

A Bombay businessman and his family used small doses (ranging from half a gram to 4 grams) of the following mixture in a spoon or dissolved in hot water to relieve digestive distress, gas, diarrhea, nausea, and vomiting:
1 part finely powdered cardamon seed
1 part finely powdered cinnamon bark
1 part finely powdered ginger root

Three single-plant diarrhea remedies

1. Tormentil (the source of tormentil red dye) rootstock (one tablespoonful of chopped rootstock steeped at least half an hour) acts astringently in cases of diarrhea; sip warm during the day. An alpine farmer told me he boiled tormentil rootstock chips in red wine to make an anti-diarrhea potion.

2. A New Delhi Indian engineer used pomegranate rind as

follows to combat the diarrhea and dysentery he suffered on his field trips: he boiled 4 ounces of the rind in 40 ounces of water until only half of the water was left, then drank at least half an ounce but no more than 2 ounces at a time. His secretary back in New Delhi used the same pomegranate remedy as a douche to clear up leukorrhea.

3. Partisans in the war-torn years around the Mediterranean chewed on grape leaves to control diarrhea, just as Colorado outdoorsmen chew on blackberry leaves for the same purpose.

Four teas to promote gallbladder and biliary function

1. Boil 1 tablespoonful of the following mixture for 2 minutes in a cupful of water 3 times a day:
   3 parts calamus root
   7 parts tumeric root

2. Decoct a tea from 1 teaspoonful of the following mixture in a cupful of water twice a day, and drink half an hour before eating:
   1 part Saint Mary's thistle foliage
   2 parts chicory root
   2 parts dandelion root

3. Brew a tea from 1 teaspoonful of the following mixture:
   1 part alder buckthorn bark
   2 part celandine foliage (poppy relative, only for experienced use. See cautions pages 42-43.)
   3 parts tumeric root
   4 parts peppermint leaves

4. Brew a tea from 1 teaspoonful of the following mixture (steep 20 minutes) 3 times a day:
   1 part caraway seeds
   1 part rhubarb root
   2 parts peppermint leaves
   2 parts Saint Benedict's thistle foliage
   2 parts Saint Mary's thistle seeds
   2 parts wormwood foliage

Stomach tea for gas, lack of appetite, and painful straining when moving bowels

Brew a tea from about 1 teaspoonful of the following mixture (Stada formula) 2 or 3 times a day:

    2 grams everlasting flowers
    5 grams valerian root
    5 grams gentian root
    5 grams calamus rhizome
    10 grams centaury foliage
    10 grams caraway seed
    10 grams aniseed
    10 grams fennel seed
    10 grams camomile flowers
    13 grams peppermint leaves
    20 grams milfoil foliage

Fresenius Four Wind Formula tea for gas, gastrocardial symptoms, swallowing of air and belching, gastrointestinal spasms, gastroenteritis (irritated mucous membranes)

Brew a tea from 1 teaspoonful (4 grams) of the following mixture:

    18.75 grams caraway seed
    25   grams aniseed
    25   grams fennel seed
    25   grams peppermint leaves
    3   grams camomile flowers
    3.25 grams Roman camomile flowers

Pour a cupful of boiling water over the teaspoonful of tea mixture and steep 5 minutes, then let it cool off to a comfortable drinking temperature. Drink a cup after each of the day's 3 main meals.

Cholangitis and cholecystitis tea

Brew a tea twice a day from about 1-2 teaspoonsful of the following mixture (Stada formula) and drink warm:

1 gram marigolds
1 gram cornflowers
5 grams gentian root
5 grams fennel seed
5 grams camomile flowers
5 grams caraway seed
8 grams restharrow root
10 grams alder buckthorn bark
10 grams celandine foliage (See cautions pages 42-43.)
20 grams peppermint leaves
30 grams dandelion root and foliage

Also as supplemental therapy for liver disease. The same precautions apply as for the other liver and gallbladder teas above.

Tea for biliary (gallbladder and ducts) irritation/irritability

Brew a tea from about 2 grams (1 filter bag) of the following mixture (Salus Chol formula) per cup:

18 grams peppermint leaves
11 grams licorice root
10 grams aniseed
10 grams Saint Benedict's thistle foliage
10 grams fennel seed
8 grams barberry rootbark
7 grams lemon balm or melissa leaves
5 grams arnica flowers (See note page 27.)
5 grams marigolds
5 grams hoarhound foliage
5 grams milfoil flowers
3 grams wormwood foliage
2 grams buckbean leaves
1 gram cornflowers

1 to 2 cups taken ½ to 1 hour before the main meals of the day.

Liver and biliary tea to prevent bile stagnation, gallstones and gravel

This tea is drunk for extended periods at 2 to 3 cups a day, each brewed by pouring 1 cupful of boiling water over 1 tablespoonful of the following mixture (Dr. Greither formula):

    5 grams artichoke leaves
    5 grams boldo leaves
    7 grams stinging nettle foliage
    6 grams mountain ash or rowan berries
    7 grams alder buckthorn bark
    3 grams fennel seed
  10 grams raspberry leaves
    4 grams camomile flowers
    3 grams purging buckthorn berries
    3 grams linseed
    7 grams linden leaves
    4 grams dandelion foliage
    4 grams everlasting flowers
    3 grams marigolds
    7 grams sage leaves
    6 grams barberries
    3 grams milfoil flowers
    8 grams juniper berries (See note page 73.)
    5 grams peppermint leaves

Don't use in cases of intestinal obstruction, and expectant mothers should be cautious. During the time when this course of tea-drinking is being followed, avoid alcohol, highly seasoned foods, and fatty meals.

Health tea to promote kidney, bladder, liver, biliary, stomach, and intestinal functions, and to prevent gas

Pour 1 cupful of boiling water over 1 tablespoonful of the following mixture (Dr. Greither formula) and steep 5 to 10 minutes (2 or 3 cups are drunk daily, each after mealtime):

    2 grams aniseed
    8 grams bearberry leaves
    7 grams blackberry leaves
    5 grams fennel

12 grams rose hips
2 grams heather
2 grams camomile flowers
5 grams coriander seeds
3 grams purging buckthorn berries
4 grams caraway
8 grams linseed
6 grams dandelion foliage
3 grams mallow flowers
3 grams peppermint leaves
3 grams marigolds
6 grams milfoil flowers
3 grams pansies
6 grams juniper berries (See note page 73.)
4 grams hawthorn leaves and flowers
8 grams horsetail foliage

Don't use in cases of intestinal obstruction, and expectant mothers should be careful.

Eleven laxative teas

(As a rule, don't rely on laxatives for more than a week at any one time; rely on diet instead.)

1. Brew a tea from 15 grams of senna leaves in 1½ quarts of water, then add 45 grams of epsom salt (magnesium sulfate). One tablespoon of this mixture in a glass of water can be taken 3 times a day.

2. Brew a tea from 7 grams of rhubarb rhizome or root in 1½ quarts of water, then add 10 grams of sodium bicarbonate (baking soda, not baking powder) plus 4 drops of peppermint oil (obtainable at gourmet and spice shops—make sure it's genuine oil and not synthetic flavoring).

3. Brew a tea from 1 teaspoonful of the following mixture:
   1 part caraway seed
   1 part orange peel
   6 parts alder buckthorn bark (inner bark from branches aged
      in storage at least a year)

4. Brew a tea from 1 teaspoonful of the following mixture:
   1 part acacia flowers (gum Arabic tree)
   1 part linden flowers
   1 part sassafras bark
   1 part senna leaves
   8 parts alder buckthorn (root) bark

5. Pour 15 parts boiling water over
   1 part roasted coffee beans (crushed) and
   1 part senna leaves
then steep 15 minutes and strain before dissolving in it:
   1 part sugar
   1 part epsom salt (magnesium sulfate)

6. Brew a tea from 1 teaspoonful of the following mixture twice a day:
   1 part aniseed
   1 part fennel seed
   6 parts senna leaves
   10 parts licorice root

7. Brew a tea from 1 teaspoonful of the following mixture:
   1 part senna leaves
   2 parts caraway seed
   3 parts alder buckthorn bark
   3 parts peppermint leaves

8. Pour 200 parts of boiling water over
   1 part chopped ginger rhizome or rootstock
   20 parts senna leaves
then steep 15 minutes and strain.

9. Brew a tea from 1 teaspoonful of the following mixture:
   1 part aniseed
   2 parts fennel seed
   2 parts licorice root
   3 parts senna leaves

10. Brew a tea from a teaspoonful of the following mixture:
   1 part elder flowers

    1   part licorice root
    1½ parts aniseed (crushed)
    1½ parts fennel seed (crushed)
    5   parts senna pods

11. Brew a tea from 1 teaspoonful of the following mixture:
    1 part fennel seed
    1 part licorice root
    2 parts peppermint leaves
    3 parts alder buckthorn bark
    3 parts senna leaves

Laxative tea

Brew a tea twice a day by pouring 1 cup of boiling water over about 1 tablespoon of the following (Stada Carilaxan formula) mixture and steeping 15 minutes:
    1   gram mallow flowers
    2   grams marigolds
    2   grams fennel seed
    2.5 grams aniseed
    4   grams pansy foliage
    5   grams elder flowers
    5   grams red sandalwood
    8.5 grams trailing bindweed flowering foliage
    10 grams restharrow root
    15 grams alder buckthorn bark
    15 grams senna leaves
    15 grams licorice root
    15 grams bean skins

For acute and chronic constipation. Don't use in cases of intestinal obstruction.

Metabolic tea

Brew a tea from 1 or 2 teaspoonsful of the following Presselin formula:
    0.5 gram cornflower
    0.5 gram marigolds

  15   grams senna leaves
  10   grams senna (Tinnevelly senna, *Cassia angustifolia*) fruit
       or pods
    7   grams fennel seed
    5   grams bean skins
    4   grams mountain ash fruit
    4   grams juniper berries (See note page 73.)
    4   grams rose hips
    2   grams everlasting flowers
  2.5 grams English daisy
  1.5 corn poppy
    3   grams camomile flowers
    2   grams blackthorn or sloe flowers
    2   grams tansy flowers (Don't take too much of tansy at once
       if you collect and mix up your own, but it's quite safe in
       professionally prepared remedies your doctor knows
       about.)
    2   grams horsetail foliage
    5   grams purging buckthorn fruit
    3   grams barberries
    5   grams couch-quitch root

For acute and chronic constipation, but don't use in cases of intestinal obstruction.

Laxative tea

Brew a tea by pouring 1 cupful of boiling water over 1 filter bag (about 1 to 2 teaspoonsful) of the following mixture (Salus-Haus formula):

   17   grams alder buckthorn bark
   13   grams caraway seed
 12.5 grams senna leaves
 12.5 grams senna pods
   11   grams licorice root
   10   grams peppermint leaves
   10   grams milfoil flowers
    7   grams pansy foliage

5   grams lemongrass
2   grams cardamom pods

Drink 1 to 2 cups morning and evening as needed for constipation and bowel movement problems in cases of hemorrhoids. Don't use in cases of intestinal obstruction.

Tea for stimulating colonic movement and the formation of bile and other digestive juices

For normalizing intestinal function when there's a tendency to constipate, 1 cupful of boiling water is poured over 1 tablespoonful of the following mixture (Dr. Greither formula) and steeped 5 to 10 minutes, preferably at bedtime:

10 grams mountain ash or rowan berries
5 grams fennel seed
8 grams camomile flowers
3 grams purging buckthorn berries
10 grams linseed
2 grams sloe, blackthorn or wild plum flowers
11 grams senna leaves
10 grams senna pods
5 grams juniper berries (See note page 73.)
7 grams horsetail foliage

Don't use in cases of intestinal obstruction, and expectant mothers should be cautious.

Hemorrhoid-relief tea

For encouraging good blood flow through the veins, firming up vessel walls, and protecting against excessive permeability of the walls, as well as easing inflammation and painful bowel movements, 3 cups of the following tea are drunk (1 cup before breakfast, 1 cup after lunch, and 1 cup before bedtime). Pour 1 cupful of boiling water over 1 tablespoon of the following mixture (Dr. Greither formula) and steep 5 to 10 minutes:

2 grams arnica flowers (See note page 27.)

4 grams camomile flowers
3 grams stinging nettle foliage
3 grams mountain ash or rowan berries
6 grams fennel seed
5 grams psyllium seed
3 grams witch hazel leaves
3 grams Saint John's wort foliage
5 grams horse chestnut leaves
3 grams mullein flowers
1 gram cornflowers
3 grams purging buckthorn berries
10 grams linseed
3 grams Saint Mary's thistle seeds
5 grams biting stonecrop or wall pepper
5 grams marigolds
10 grams milfoil flowers
6 grams senna leaves
6 grams senna pods
7 grams knotgrass foliage
7 grams horsetail foliage

Don't use in cases of intestinal obstruction, and expectant mothers should be cautious.

Slenderizing tea

Brew a tea 1 to 3 times a day from about 1 teaspoonful of the following mixture (Hameln Antiviscosin formula):
28 grams senna leaves
28 grams alder buckthorn bark
10 grams aniseed
9 grams fennel seed
9 grams milfoil foliage
9 grams couch-quitch root
7 grams bladder wrack

For obesity, gastrointestinal upsets, lazy bowels, tendency to accumulate fat. Don't use in cases of intestinal obstruction, sensitivity to iodine (which is, by the way, contained in the bladder wrack), thyrotoxicosis, decompensated cardiac insufficiency or tuberculosis.

Tea to prevent nutritional obesity in people who lack exercise and who tend to constipate

Pour 1 cupful of boiling water over 1 tablespoonful of the following mixture (Dr. Greither formula) and steep 5 to 10 minutes; 2 to 3 cups a day are drunk.

4 grams aniseed
10 grams birch leaves
4 grams watercress foliage
7 grams alder buckthorn bark
3 grams fennel seed
5 grams lemongrass
2 grams caraway seed
2 grams parsley fruit or "seed"
6 grams milfoil flowers
2 grams celery fruit or "seed"
8 grams senna leaves
10 grams senna pods
6 grams juniper berries (See note page 73.)
2 grams water fennel seed
9 grams horsetail foliage

Don't use in cases of intestinal obstruction, and expectant mothers should be cautious.

Section 7

Combination Anti-Diabetic Teas

The Dr. Greither Formula diabetic tea is drunk daily in the place of other beverages, without sugar, to support medical therapy of diabetes; it is not meant to replace any insulin being prescribed by a physician. Besides their favorable effect on people who suffer from diabetes, these plants also encourage good urinary and gastrointestinal function. Pour 1 cupful of boiling water over 1 tablespoonful of the following mixture and steep 5 to 10 minutes:

6 grams birch leaves
1 gram buckbean leaves
10 grams bladder wrack
10 grams bean skins
8 grams stinging nettle foliage
2 grams fennel seed
5 grams galega or goat's rue foliage
8 grams blueberry leaves
4 grams hibiscus flower bases
5 grams hops
2 grams cornflowers
2 grams caraway
5 grams European mistletoe foliage (See note page 84·)
5 grams orange blossoms
10 grams couch-quitch rootstock
10 grams hawthorn flowers and leaves
7 grams horsetail foliage

The Kühne formula diabetic tea to support the medical treatment of diabetes, particularly senile diabetes, is brewed by pouring 1 cupful of boiling water over 1 teaspoonful to 1 tablespoonful of the following mixture and steeping 5 to 10 minutes; this tea is drunk as desired during the day:

17.4 parts blackberry leaves

4.4 parts strawberry leaves
1.8 parts seedless rose hips
3.6 parts raspberry leaves
0.4 part cornflowers
1.8 parts linden flowers
1.8 parts peppermint leaves
0.9 part marigolds
3.6 parts woodruff foliage
25   parts blueberry leaves
25   parts bean skins
1.8 parts boldo leaves
7.1 parts oat straw
1.8 parts tormentil root
3.6 parts juniper berries (See note page 73.)

Note the large amounts of blueberry leaves and bean skins, both known for their favorable effect on diabetes.

The Ikabo formula diabetic tea is brewed by pouring 1 cupful of boiling water over 1 tablespoon of the mixture given below, steeping it 30 minutes before straining out the plant parts. Some Europeans use sweeteners in this tea, of which they drink only 2 cups a day at first, then later drink as many as 3 to 4 cups a day. It is recommended that the whole amount be drunk in the morning.

21 grams blueberry leaves
 9 grams boldo leaves
 9 grams field poppies
 9 grams mallow flowers
 5 grams blackberry leaves
14 grams linseed
20 grams bean skins
 4 grams marigold flowers
 9 grams everlasting flowers

The Mauermann formula diabetic tea for supplemental therapy is brewed as usual from 1 tablespoon of the following mixture.

25 grams blueberry leaves
10 grams boldo leaves

10 grams rosemary leaves
10 grams stinging nettle leaves
10 grams bearberry leaves
 5 grams marigold flowers
20 grams galega (goat's rue) foliage
10 grams linseed

Seven combination diabetic teas

Plant and parts

	Bean skins	Bearberry leaves	Birch leaves	Blueberry leaves	Buckthorn bark	Dandelion foliage and root	Galega foliage	Galega seeds	Lady's mantle foliage	Pansy foliage	Peppermint leaves	Stinging nettle foliage	Valerian root
1.	*			*					*				
2.	*			*		*	*						
3.		*		*			*						*
4.			*	*	*		*						
5.	*			*			*			*			
6.	*		*	*								*	
7.	*			*			*	*			*		

Proportion and remarks

1:2:1.	
1:2:1.	
2:3:3:2.	3 or 4 cups a day, 1 cup before each meal for any of these five teas
1:4:1:4.	
Equal parts of each.	

1:2:6:1. Bring to a boil. 2 or 3 cups a day

Equal parts of each. 1 cup boiling water over 1 tablespoonful and steep 15-20 minutes. 3 or 4 cups a day.

Section 8

Combination Teas
to Alleviate
Genito-Urinary Distress

Seven teas to promote urinary flow

1. Brew a tea from 1 teaspoonful of the following mixture:
   1 part fennel seed
   1 part licorice root
   3 parts juniper berries

Note: Because of the juniper berries in this remedy, it is not recommended for use by persons suffering from acute kidney inflammation or during pregnancy.

2. Brew a tea from 1 teaspoonful of the following mixture:
   1 part juniper berries (See note, Tea 1 above.)
   1 part licorice root
   1 part parsley root
   1 part restharrow root

3. Brew a tea from 1 teaspoonful of the following mixture (by soaking it several hours in 1 cup of cold water and then boiling it for 10 to 20 minutes):
   1 part juniper berries (See note, Tea 1.)
   1 part licorice root
   1 part lovage root
   1 part restharrow root

4. Brew a tea from 1 teaspoonful of the following mixture (by soaking and boiling as for the preceding tea):
   1 part asparagus root

1 part coughgrass root
1 part licorice root
1 part marshmallow root
1 part strawberry root

Asparagus (which contains saponin, tannin, potassium salts, asparagin, and other amino acids) encourages the flow or urine, especially of its chlorine and phosphate components. On rare occasions, some people have shown some allergic reaction to asparagus, and it shouldn't be used as a remedy in case of kidney disease.

5. Brew a tea by pouring a pint of boiling water over 1 heaped teaspoonful of the following mixture:
   1 part Indian kidney tea leaves
   1 part maté leaves
   2 parts bean skins
   2 parts bearberry leaves
   2 parts birch leaves
   2 parts horsetail foliage

6. Brew a tea from 1 teaspoonful of the following mixture:
   1   part licorice root
   1   part milfoil foliage
   1½ part birch leaves
   2   parts juniper berries (See note page 180.)
   2   parts restharrow root
   2½ parts parsley root

7. Brew a tea from 1 teaspoonful of the following mixture:
   1 part aniseed
   1 part parsley seed
   2 parts pansy foliage
   4 parts juniper berries (See note page 180.)
   4 parts licorice root
   4 parts lovage root
   4 parts restharrow root

Bladder tea

Brew a tea from 1 teaspoonful of the following mixture:

1 part birch leaves
1 part bearberry leaves
1 part rupturewort foliage

Antimicrobial bladder tea

Brew a tea from 1 teaspoonful of the following mixture:
    3 parts couchgrass root or rhizome
    4 parts birch leaves
    5 parts licorice root
    8 parts bearberry leaves

To add a cramp-relieving effect to the above remedy, European physicians have added 2 parts of henbane or poison tobacco (*Hyoscyamus niger*) to it—but this is mentioned here only as an illustration of how remedies are composed, and is *not* recommended for home use. Henbane is one of the plants—a poisonous one—best left to experienced physicians with herbal knowledge.

Bladder and kidney tea for supplemental therapy for acute and chronic cystitis, pyelitis and kidney stones

Brew a tea 3 times a day by pouring 1 pint of boiling water over about 1 tablespoonful of the following mixture (Stada formula) and steeping it 15 minutes before straining out the plant parts:
    1 gram marigolds
    4 grams red sandalwood
    5 grams asparagus root
    10 grams goldenrod foliage
    10 grams Indian kidney tea leaves
    10 grams peppermint leaves
    10 grams bean skins
    10 gram horsetail foliage
    10 grams rupturewort foliage
    15 grams bearberry leaves
    15 grams birch leaves

Tea for kidney stones, nephritis, cystitis pyelitis, dropsy, and bacteriuria (bacteria in the urine)

Brew a tea 3 times a day from about 1 teaspoonful of the following mixture (Mauermann Nephronorm formula):

   10 grams heather flowers
    5 grams broom flowers
    5 grams birch leaves
    5 grams boldo leaves
    5 grams Indian kidney tea leaves
   15 grams bearberry leaves
    5 grams juniper berries (See note page 180.)
    5 grams rupturewort foliage
    5 grams goldenrod foliage
    5 grams restharrow root
   30 grams madder root

To simplify formulas like this one that have a convenient common denominator (5 in this case), divide everything by 5, giving you 2 grams of heather instead of 10 grams, 1 gram of broom instead of 5 grams, and so on.

Tea for uric acid problems, acute and chronic kidney and bladder ailments, dropsy

Pour 1 cupful of boiling water over 1 teaspoonful of the following mixture (Vogel & Weber Nephrubin formula), steep 10 minutes before straining; drink 1 cupful, a mouthful at a time, in the morning and 1 cupful in the evening:

   7.5 grams willow bark
   7.5 grams horsechestnut flowers
   7.5 grams elder flowers
   7.5 grams linden flowers
   7.5 grams birch leaves
   7.5 grams parsley seed
   7.5 grams rupturewort foliage
   7 5 grams guaiac wood
   7.5 grams celery root
   25 grams Indian kidney tea leaves

Tea for inflammation of the urethra, bladder, ureters, and kidney pelvis (the kidney cavity from which the ureter exits)

Brew a tea 3 times a day from 2 teaspoonsful (per cup) of the following mixture (Hoyer Nieron formula):

1 part bean skins
1 part birch leaves
1 part bearberry leaves
1 part horsetail foliage
1 part rupturewort foliage
1 part dandelion root and foliage
1 part eryngo foliage
1 part restharrow root
1 part linseed

Diuretic as supplementary therapy for urinary infections

Brew a tea 2 or 3 times a day from 2 grams (per cup of water) of the following mixture (Salus Uron formula):

10 grams birch leaves
10 grams rupturewort foliage
10 grams juniper berries (See note page 180.)
10 grams milfoil flowers
10 grams Indian kidney tea leaves
10 grams red sandalwood
10 grams punarnava leaves
 8 grams bearberry leaves
 7 grams fennel seed
 7 grams parsley seed
 5 grams horsetail foliage
 3 grams bucco leaves

Two teas for healthy urinary organs

Plants in the tea	Dr. Greither formula 23 to strengthen and stimulate the kidneys and the bladder	Dr. Greither formula 29 to encourage urinary flow
Bearberry leaves	12 grams	13 grams
Birch leaves	13 grams	16 grams
Goldenrod foliage	7 grams	none
Rose hips seeds	6 grams	8 grams
Blueberry leaves	9 grams	none
Heather flowers	6 grams	7 grams
Indian kidney tea	6 grams	none
Parsley seed	4 grams	1 gram
Celery seed	3 grams	none
Juniper berries	6 grams	8 grams
Horsetail foliage	7 grams	7 grams
Lemongrass	none	5 grams
Rosemary leaves	none	8 grams
Blackthorn, sloe or wild plum	none	3 grams
Hawthorn flowers and leaves	none	10 grams
Hawthorn berries	none	1 gram
	To prepare either tea, pour 1 cupful of boiling water over 1 tablespoonful of either of the above mixture.	
	Formula 23 is drunk at meals.	Formula 29 is sipped slowly, 1 cup before breakfast, and 1 cup in late afternoon. Don't use in cases of kidney or heart disease.

Tea to improve kidney and bladder function, increase urinary flow, and help against cystitis

Brew a tea from 1 heaping tablespoonful of the following mixture (Galama formula) for each cup of water:

    15 grams bearberry leaves
    13 grams birch leaves
    10 grams rose hips
     9 grams juniper berries (See note page 180.)
     5 grams everlasting
    11 grams horsetail foliage
     4 grams rosemary leaves
     2 grams mallow flowers
    10 grams restharrow root
     6 grams bean skins
     3 grams Indian kidney tea
     2 grams rupturewort foliage

Section 9

Combination Teas and Rinses
to Alleviate Women's Conditions

Astringent, anti-inflammatory, deodorant,
and anti-cramping vaginal douches

Douches have been prepared from various combinations of blackberry leaves, camomile flowers, crampweed (silverweed) foliage, lady's mantle, lavender flowers, mallow flowers, meadowsweet, milfoil foliage, oak bark (inner), rosemary leaves, sage leaves, thyme foliage, walnut leaves, white nettle (or blind nettle, dead nettle) and other plants. Here are three simple two-plant combinations which have been used to alleviate leukorrhea, vulvitis, vaginitis, malodorous conditions, and cramps:

	Douche 1	Douche 2	Douche 3 Aromatic deodorant
1 part camomile flowers	*	*	
1 part crampweed foliage	*		
1 part lavender flowers			*
1 part sage leaves		*	
1 part thyme foliage			*

To prepare douches 1 and 2, pour 1 quart of boiling water over about 5 teaspoonsful of the above mixtures.

Pour 1 quart of boiling water over about 2 teaspoonsful of the above mixture and steep 15 minutes.

Use about twice a day as needed. Avoid excessive, long-term use of sage and thyme.

187

Three women's teas for regulating menstruation

1. Brew a tea from 1 teaspoonful of the following mixture·
   1 part alder buckthorn bark
   1 part couchgrass root
   1 part milfoil foliage
   1 part senna leaves

2. Brew a tea from 1 teaspoonful of the following mixture (by boiling several minutes in one cupful of water):
   1   part alder buckthorn bark
   1½ part lemon balm or melissa leaves
   1½ part valerian root
   10   parts crampweed foliage
Drink about 4 cups a day just before the menstrual period is expected, and also when it begins.

3. Brew a tea from 1 tablespoonful of the following mixture (by pouring half a pint of boiling water over it and steeping 5 minutes in a covered container):
   1 part alder buckthorn
   1 part birch leaves
   1 part blackberry leaves and foliage
   1 part heather flowering shoots
   2 parts milfoil foliage
   2 parts peppermint leaves
   2 parts valerian root
Drink a cup or two hot daily.

The Klimax-Fink formula tea for climacteric symptoms, constipation and gas is brewed from a teaspoonful of the following mixture:
   25   grams fennel seed
   22.5 grams senna leaves
   30   grams couch-quitch root
   22.5 grams licorice root
Caution should be used with this tea during pregnancy.

Vogel & Weber Echtroklim formula tea for pre-menopausal and menopausal problems is brewed by pouring 1 cupful of boiling water over 2 teaspoonsful of the following mixture and steeping 10 minutes before straining; drink at mealtimes, up to 2 or 3 cups a day:

- 6 grams crampweed foliage
- 6 grams wormwood foliage
- 6 grams woodruff foliage
- 7 grams goldenrod foliage
- 6 grams red sandalwood
- 16 grams chinese yellow berry buds
- 10 grams sloe-leaf viburnum, highbush cranberry, or crampbark
- 10 grams milfoil flowers
- 6 grams lemon balm or melissa leaves
- 15 grams hawthorn leaves
- 6 grams peppermint leaves
- 6 grams lady's mantle foliage

Section 10

Combination Teas That
Settle the Nerves and Promote Sleep

Ten nerve-soothing teas

1. Brew a tea from 1 teaspoonful of the following mixture:
    1 part lemon balm or melissa leaves
    1 part peppermint leaves
    2 parts valerian root
Put the valerian root fragments in the cold water, bring to a boil, then add the boiling water to the melissa and peppermint leaves, and steep 5 or 10 minutes.

2. Brew a tea from 2 teaspoonsful of the following mixture (by soaking in a cup of cold water 30 minutes then bringing to a boil for 3 minutes):
    1 part hops (female catkins)
    1 part orange leaves
    2 parts valerian root

3. Brew a tea from a teaspoonful of the following mixture:
    3 parts buckbean leaves
    3 parts valerian root
    2 parts orange peel
Drink a cup or two at night.

4. Brew a tea from 2 teaspoonsful of the following mixture:
    1   part lemon balm or melissa leaves
    1   part valerian root
    2½ parts hops catkeins

5. Brew a tea from 2 teaspoonsful of the following mixture (by pouring a cupful of boiling water over it and steeping 5 minutes).

1 part buckbean leaves
1 part orange leaves (or flowers)
1 part peppermint leaves
1 part valerian root
Drink 1 cupful slowly an hour before bed.

6. Brew a tea from a teaspoonful of the following mixture:
    1 part lemon balm or melissa leaves
    1 part peppermint leaves
    1 part orange blossoms
    1 part bitter orange peel (*Citrus aurantium.* You can also use
        sweet orange, *Citrus sinensis*, although its effect is weaker.)
    6 parts valerian root

7. Brew a tea from a teaspoonful of the following mixture:
    1   part lemon balm or melissa leaves
    1   part peppermint leaves
    1½ parts aniseed (crushed)
    2   parts orange blossoms
    2   parts passionflower foliage
    2½ parts valerian root

8. Brew a tea from 2 teaspoonsful of the following Stada formula
mixture (by pouring 1 cupful of boiling water over it and steeping 15
minutes in a covered container):
    1 part marigolds
    5 parts hops catkins
    10 parts peppermint leaves
    10 parts rosemary leaves
    15 parts blackberry leaves
    15 parts Saint John's wort foliage
    20 parts lemon balm leaves
    24 parts valerian root
Drink 2 or 3 cups a day.

9. Brew a tea from 1 teaspoonful of the following mixture:
    1 part lavender flowers
    1 part marjoram

1 part peppermint leaves
1 part rosemary leaves
1 part roses
1 part thyme foliage
1 part wild marjoram or oregano foliage
1 part wild thyme foliage

10. The Agrimonas formula nerve tea is brewed from a teaspoonful of the following mixture per cupful of water; 1 or 2 cups are drunk daily:

2 grams citrus rind
3 grams larkspur flowers
2 grams marigolds
2 grams lavender flowers
4 grams mallow flowers
8 grams lemon balm or melissa leaves
5 grams rosemary leaves
8 grams caraway seeds
12 grams fennel seeds
8 grams crampweed or silverweed foliage
2 grams centaury foliage
17 grams Saint John's wort foliage
18 grams peppermint leaves
2 grams licorice root
2.68 grams hops

Four teas to overcome nervous insomnia

1. The Kühne formula tea to relax nerves and combat insomnia is brewed by pouring 1 cupful of boiling water over 1 tablespoonful of the following mixture, steeping a few minutes. Drink it before going to bed:

15.5   parts blackberry leaves
3.9   parts strawberry leaves
4.7   parts rose hips (without seeds)
3.1   parts raspberry leaves
0.4   parts cornflower
1.5   parts linden flowers

1.5   parts peppermint leaves
0.8   parts marigolds
6.3   parts woodruff foliage
1.5   parts valerian root
9.4   parts heather flowers
9.4   parts Saint John's wort foliage
3.1   parts lemon balm or melissa leaves
3.1   parts European mistletoe foliage (See note page 84.)
1.5   parts rosemary leaves
3.1   parts milfoil foliage
3.1   parts hawthorn flowers, leaves, stems
3.1   parts horsetail foliage
3.1   parts juniper berries (See note page 180.)
1.88 parts hops
3.1   parts lavender flowers

2. The Ikabo formula nerve and sleep tea is brewed by pouring 1 cupful of boiling water over 1 tablespoonful of the following mixture and steeping 30 minutes before straining out plant parts:

13 grams lemon balm or melissa leaves
13 grams orange blossoms
13 grams cowslip or primrose flowers
 7 grams corn poppy
 7 grams hops
13 grams lavender flowers
13 grams heather flowers
14 grams Saint John's wort foliage
 7 grams larkspur flowers

Sweeten to taste. A cup is drunk at bedtime, or during the day if needed to calm overexcitement.

3. Dr. Greither formula tea for nervous, tense and excited conditions of functional and psychic origin is brewed by pouring 1 cupful of boiling water over 1 tablespoonful of the following mixture to make 1 cup of nerve tea (drink 2 cups a day); for insomnia, the tea is drunk an hour before bedtime:

4   grams camomile flowers
5   grams birch leaves

7   grams dill seed
3   grams fumitory foliage
8   grams fennel seed
.3   grams wild or English daisy
5.33 grams heather flowers
6   grams elderberries
7   grams hops
4   grams Saint John's foliage
3.33 grams everlasting flowers
6.67 grams night-blooming cereus flowers
7   grams lavender flowers
5   grams lemon balm or melissa leaves
4   grams peony (See note page 135.)
6   grams orange blossoms
6.67 grams rosemary leaves
4   grams woundwort or kidney vetch
         flowers
5   grams horsetail foliage

4. Salus Dorm formula tea for nervous excitation, insomnia, heart is brewed from 2 grams of the following mixture per cup (1 cup taken in the morning and 1 or 2 before retiring for the night):

10 grams passionflower foliage
10 grams peppermint leaves
10 grams hawthorn flowers and leaves
10 grams lemon balm (melissa) leaves
10 grams coriander seed
 8 grams valerian root
 8 grams lavender flowers
 8 grams orange blossoms
 6 grams jatamansi root
 6 grams hollow root (corydalis rootstock)
 6 grams hops catkins
 6 grams dill seed
 2 grams cinnamon bark

Section 11

Combination Remedies
for Skin and Foot Conditions

Seven-plant wet dressing for skin
problems in general

Brew a tea from a teaspoonful of the following mixture and apply it warm or cool several times a day:
    1 part lemon balm or melissa leaves
    1 part marjoram foliage
    1 part oregano or wild marjoram foliage
    1 part peppermint leaves
    1/3 part camomile flowers
    1/3 part elder flowers
    1/3 part lavender flowers

If you've noted that certain mixtures or individual plants seem to provide more relief than others for your particular condition and needs, then a little careful experimentation could lead to just the right remedy for you. For example, if you note that combinations with camomile relieve your inflammation better, then try that alone, or add more of it to the recipe. Be cautions, though, for some plants or their parts may be too strong alone (some kinds of senna, for example, may cause griping when taken alone), or may not develop their best properties unless mixed with other plants. Unless you're an experienced botanist, don't attempt to go out into the woods and look for plants that seem similar to the ones that you've used in the kitchen for relief. Even the right plant at the wrong time can be unpleasant, such as fresh buckthorn bark, which must be heated or stored for a year before it loses its nauseating properties.

Fourteen combination external soaks, baths, and cataplasms for alleviating inflamed skin conditions

Plant and parts

Recipe	Angelica root	Arnica flowers	Calamus rhizome	Camomile flowers	Comfrey root	Flax (linseed)	Goldenrod foliage	Heather foliage	Horsetail foliage	Lavender flowers	Mallow flowers	Mallow leaves	Marigolds	Marshmallow leaves
1.				*							*			
2.			*											
3.	*		*											
4.														
5.														
6.		*		*										
7.					*	*							*	
8.		*		*					*					
9.							*	*	*					
10.														
11.				*										
12.										*				
13.		*		*						*				
14.				*		*						*		*

Melilot foliage	Oak inner bark	Mullein flowers	Pansy foliage	Rosemary leaves	Thyme foliage	Tormentil rhizome	Walnut leaves	Willow inner bark	Proportions and remarks
									Equal parts
	*								Equal parts
									Equal parts
	*					*			Equal parts. Boil 10 minutes
			*			*			Equal parts. Boil 3 minutes. Steep 10 minutes. Change wet dressing every ½ hour for runny eczema.
									Equal parts
									4:3:3. Apply cool or body temperature on leg ulcers or poorly healing sores.
									3:3:4
									4:3:3 on poorly healing wounds
	*					*		*	3:3:4. Soak 1-2 tablespoonsful in cupful of cold water several hours, then boil 10 minutes. For poorly healing wounds and abscesses
		*	*						2:2:1
				*	*			*	1:1:1:7. For rheumatism as well as skin inflammation
				*	*				6:6:1:1:6. Pour 1 pint boiling water over 1-2 tablespoonsful. Steep a few minutes and apply lukewarm.
*									Equal parts

Hibiscus and peach poultice for itching, burning blisters

For easing the symptoms of pemphigus (an itching, burning blistering condition, the causes of which require a physician's services), a Hong Kong jeweler applied a poultice made from peach leaves mashed in vinegar plus mashed up fresh hibiscus (*Hibiscus mutabilis*) flowers.

Note: Peach kernels, by the way, were used by the ancient Egyptians the way the Ancient Greeks used poison hemlock—as an official execution potion. The kernels of peaches and related species, especially bitter almonds, contain hydrocyanic acid.

Footbaths for tired, aching, cold, and sweaty feet

The waiter who brought me my coffee, beer, and open-faced sandwiches the day I trekked eight hours over Tyrolean hills and Alpine meadows near Bad Reichenhall, explained how he bathed his sweaty, tired, burning feet for fifteen minutes a day in a footbath of dwarf pine needles, rosemary leaves and salt (from natural mineral brine)—a formula he learned from a friend who worked at a nearby firm (Josef-Mack) that manufactures ready-made capsules of that mix (called La-Ro-Sol).

A Hong King shoe salesman who saved money by making do with odd-sized shoes that never really fit his feet, softened his corns and alleviated the aches they caused him by soaking his feet nightly in a "tea" he made by boiling fresh turnip leaves and pink radish leaves. Sometimes he added a little alum, too, to intensify the footbath's effect. A week's treatment would have been sufficient for many of his aching corns, but he often kept right on squeezing his feet into poorly fitting shoes, which, of course, kept encouraging the formation and growth of his painful corns. (See Section 2 for how a Japanese bus driver relieved swollen testicles with the same two vegetables—turnips and radishes.)

The following table explains eight other footbaths:

Condition	Plant	How to use
Tired, flat feet	Horsetail foliage	Brew handful of foliage in one pint of water.
Gangrenous sores Rheumatic stiffness	Male fern. Also an ancient tapeworm remedy, but its poisonous properties limit its use here only to an external footbath.	Boil one pound of rootstock in vinegar and add to footbath.
Gout	Male fern	Boil one pound of rootstock in water and add to footbath. Bathe every few days for a week or so (according to a Swiss farmer).
Perspiration	Couchgrass, lady's mantle, oak bark	Brew a handful of lady's mantle foliage in one quart of water. Or boil down a handful of either couchgrass rhizome or oak inner bark in one quart of water until one pint of liquid remains, then add to the footbath.
Weak feet	Willow inner bark, yellow gentian root	Boil a handful of bark or root in one quart of water, and add to footbath (about a quart of either hot or cold water). Use frequently.
Cold or tired feet	Oat straw	Boil a pound or two of oat straw in 3 quarts or so of water for half an hour. Dilute if necessary before soaking feet in it.

Section 12

Combination Spring Cures for Healthy Blood, Skin, and Physiology

Some people might think that "spring cures" are uselessly old-fashioned and that "cleansing and purifying the blood" is a claim made by wild west medicine shows. There is hardly anything as far from the truth as that view. Other people admit that spring cures were once needed to catch up once a year on all the lack of fresh fruits and vegetables they missed during each long, hard winter, but not today, they think, when deep freezes and other technology bring us anything anytime anywhere. Wrong again, for the availability of good foods today is often obscured by a just-as-overwhelming availability of unworthy foods (and food substitutes!). And many of us overindulge in them. So we still have a pressing need to cleanse out the system. But cleansing and purifying the system (that is, the tissues, one of which is the blood that carries nutrients throughout us) is also important for another reason besides helping us to deal with poor diets and eating habits. It's important because it gives us a way to get at stubborn skin and other chronic conditions *from the inside*. That is especially important for persons who are predisposed to skin and membrane inflammations.

1. Here's an **Austrian tea** from roots and wood (boil 2 tablespoonsful of chopped pieces or shavings in 3 cupsful of water down to 2 cups to get the ingredients out of the wood):
1 part burdock root
1 part licorice root

1 part red sandalwood
1 part sarsaparilla root
2 parts guaiac wood
2 parts juniper twigs (See note page 73.)
2 parts sassafras rootbark or wood
1 or 2 cupfuls are drunk warm for breakfast.

2. Here's another **blood purifying tea** of which 2 or 3 cups are drunk during the day. For each cupful, boil a tablespoonful or so of the following mixture for about 3 minutes in a cupful of water:
1 part crushed fennel seed
1 part licorice root
2 parts alder buckthorn bark
2 parts birch leaves
2 parts elder flowers
2 parts pansy foliage

Blood and system purification, of course, may involve increased sweat and urine excretion, and, as you can see from the buckthorn ingredient, also some laxative effect.

3. **The Agrimonas formula tea** is brewed by pouring a cupful of boiling water over 1 teaspoonful of the following mixture; 1 to 2 cups are drunk morning and evening for extended periods.
5 grams alder buckthorn bark
2 grams orange peel
3 grams orange blossoms
3 grams larkspur (See note page 135.)
1 gram marigolds
3 grams mallow flowers
2 grams everlasting flowers
12 grams birch leaves
6 grams walnut leaves
9 grams senna leaves
10 grams caraway seeds
12 grams fennel seeds
9 grams crampweed foliage

1 gram centaury foliage
5 grams red sandalwood
2 grams licorice root
3 grams hops
2.68 grams restharrow root

4. **The Galama formula tea** is brewed from a heaping tablespoon of the following mixture and drunk over extended periods not only as a laxative, but also for its blood-cleansing effect:

5 grams hibiscus flowers
5 grams camomile flowers
5 grams elder flowers
5 grams everlasting flowers
6 grams birch leaves
6 grams walnut leaves
5 grams peppermint leaves
11 grams senna leaves
7 grams senna pods
4 grams stinging nettle foliage
5 grams caraway seeds
4 grams fennel seeds
6 grams fumitory flowering plant
9 grams milfoil foliage
4 grams guaiac wood
6 grams sandalwood
5 grams restharrow root

5. **The Dr. Greither formula tea** is brewed by pouring 1 cupful of boiling water over 1 heaping tablespoonful of the following mixture, and drunk to stimulate the excretion of metabolic wastes from the intestines, kidneys and skin; expectant mothers should use care, and don't use in cases of intestinal obstruction:

6 grams birch leaves
8 grams alder buckthorn bark
3 grams fennel seeds
10 grams rose hips

5 grams heather flowers and/or flowering shoots
2 grams coriander seeds
3 grams caraway seeds
8 grams linseed
2 grams Saint Mary's thistle seeds
3 grams celery seeds
4 grams senna fruit
7 grams senna pods
4 grams milfoil flowers
3 grams cowslip or primrose flowers
8 grams juniper berries (See note page 180.)
3 grams walnut leaves

Appendix

Laboratories and Firms That Supply Plant Parts, Ready-Made Teas, Tinctures, Elixers, Tablets, Oils, Baths, and Tonics Made from Plants

Below are the names and addresses of the firms and laboratories which kindly responded to my requests for detailed technical information on their medicinal teas and other products, especially those mentioned in the right column.

A. Niedermeier Chem.-pharm. Fabrik Taufkirchner Strasse 59 8011 Hohenbrunn West Germany	Agrimonas formula teas, etc.
Bio-Diät-Berlin Karlsruher Strasse 7a-8 1 Berlin 31 West Germany	Kühne formula teas, etc.
Cernelle AB Vegelholm 6250 Engelholm Sweden	Pollen extract, vitamins, minearals, and proteins in tablets, ointments, etc.
Cernitin S.A. P.O. Box 234 6903 Lugano Switzerland	Pollen extract, vitamins, minerals, and proteins in tablets, ointments, etc.

Dibona KG Postfach 1253 D-7505 Ettlingen West Germany	Honey from a variety of forest, flower, and meadow types
Dr. Dünner Kirschberghauserstrasse 35 9533 Sankt Gallen Switzerland	Bran, pollen, herbal tablets
Dr. E. Fresenius Pharma Borkenberg 14 6370 Oberursel/Taunus 1 West Germany	Four-Wind and other teas, etc.
Dr. Otto Greither	*See* Salus-Haus *further below*
Floradix fruit extract and iron tonic	*See* Salus-Haus *further below*
Galama	*See* Hayo Folkerts *further below*
General Nutrition Corporation 921 Penn Avenue Pittsburgh, PA, 15222	General line of health items, especially products low in salt, sugar and fats
Hoyer Co. Postfach 1240 4040 Neuss 21 West Germany	Galema formula teas, etc.
Ikabo-Kräuterhaus J. Kneider Postfach 1365 4630 Bochum West Germany	Teas
Johann Georg Fink Co. Daimlerstrasse 3 7033 Herrenberg West Germany	Teas, etc.
Josef Mack KG Innsbrucker Strasse 37 8230 Bad Reichenhall West Germany	Herbal foot baths, arnica, evergreen remedies, etc.

Key West Aloe Company Key West, Florida	Aloe extracts
Mauermann-Arzneimittel 8134 Pocking-Starnberger See West Germany	Teas, etc.
Nam Kwong Trading Company Nan Tung Bank Building Rua da Praia Grande, 65-A Macao	Ginseng, etc.
Penn Herb Co. Ltd. 603 North 2nd Street Philadelphia, PA 19123	Teas, health items
Pharma Hameln Postfach 2456 3250 Hameln 1 (Afferde) West Germany	Teas, etc. (Hameln, by the way, is the town where the Pied Piper led the mice, rats ... and children out of town and disappeared into a mountain!)
Po-Ho-Co (Olbas) Grellingerstrasse 40 Basle, Switzerland	Mixtures of ethereal oils (Basle or Po-Ho oil)
Presselin-Werk GmbH & Co Postfach 1346 4983 Kirchlengern I.W. West Germany	Teas, etc.
Ricola Ltd. CH-4242 Laufen Switzerland	Swiss herbal candy and tea
Roth & Son 1577 First Avenue New York, NY 10028	Spices, seasonings, herbal teas, etc.
Salus of America 250 Newport Center Drive 207 Newport Beach, California 92660	Most of Salus-Haus items
Salus-Haus Bahnhofstrasse 24 8206 Bruckmühl/Mangfall West Germany	Teas, Bavarian herbal bonbons, elixirs, baths, etc.

Stada Arzneimittel AG Stada-Strasse 2-18 6368 Bad Vilbel 4 West Germany	Teas, etc.
Teck Soon Hong, Ltd. 37 Connaught Road, W. Teck Soon Building Hong Kong	Ginseng, etc.
Vogel & Weber GmbH Herrschinger Strasse 33 8084 Inning/Ammersee West Germany	Teas, etc.
W. Atlee Burpee Seed Co. Fordhook Farms Doylestown, PA 18901	Seeds
Weleda AG Stollenrain 11 4144 Arlesheim Switzerland	Herbal remedies and cosmetics, etc.

Index of Plants, Their Uses, and Health Problems

In addition to these page numbers, plants are mentioned on other pages, particularly in combination recipes in Sections 4 to 12.

Upper respiratory infections and inflammations (*cont.*)
(*see also* Colds and "flu")
Urinary tract conditions, 31, 33, 64, 77,
92, 98, 102, 119, 133, 180-186

Vaginal discharge (leukorrhea), 100
Valerian (*Valeriana officinalis*), 116,
128
Varicose veins, 129, 134
Venous problems, 67, 129
Violet (*Viola odorata*), 117
Violetroot or poison hay (*Iris germanica*),
143
Vitamins, 32, 33, 47, 54, 58, 65, 93, 99,
101, 112, 113
Volatile oils, (*see* Ethereal oils)

Walnut (*Juglans regia*, etc.), 142

Warts, 42, 91, 114, 122, 123
Watercress (*Nasturtium officinale*), 87
Wheat germ, 127
Willow (*Salix alba*), 97
Wine, 62
Wintergreen (*Gaultheria procumbens*),
98
Witch hazel (*Hamamelis virginica*),
117-118
Woodruff (*Asperula odorata*), 156
Wormwood (*Artemisia absinthium*), 126
Wounds and sores, 22, 42, 56, 61, 70,
74, 80, 85, 95, 104, 113, 114,
118-121, 195-197

Xanthophyll, 112

Yeast (*Saccharomyces* species), 127